Dash Diet Cookbook for Beginners

Low Sodium Cookbook Recipes to Lower Blood Pressure and Improve Your Health that You Can Prep Fast

Claudia Rivera

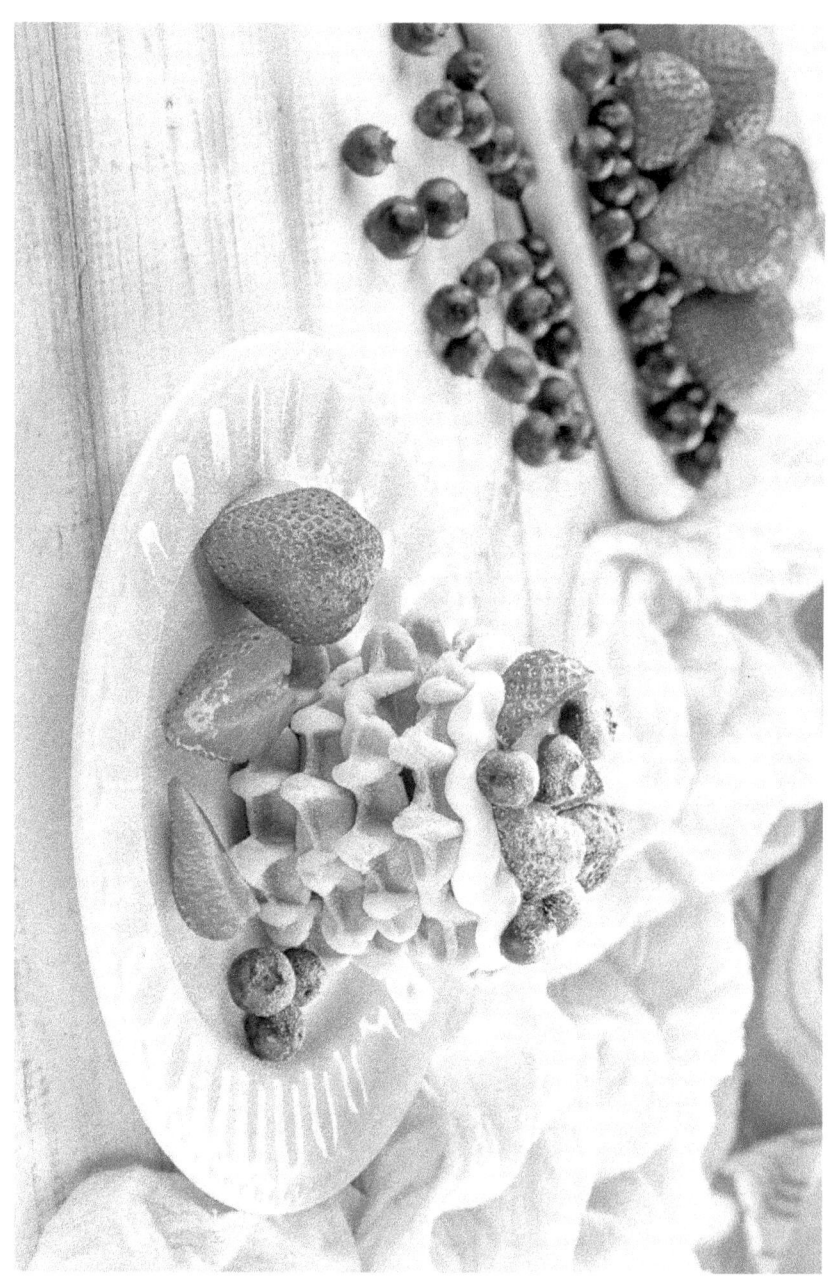

© Copyright 2020 by Claudia Rivera - All rights reserved.

The following Book is reproduced below with the goal of providing information that is as accurate and reliable as possible. Regardless, purchasing this Book can be seen as consent to the fact that both the publisher and the author of this book are in no way experts on the topics discussed within and that any recommendations or suggestions that are made herein are for entertainment purposes only. Professionals should be consulted as needed prior to undertaking any of the action endorsed herein.

This declaration is deemed fair and valid by both the American Bar Association and the Committee of Publishers Association and is legally binding throughout the United States.

Furthermore, the transmission, duplication, or reproduction of any of the following work including specific information will be considered an illegal act irrespective of if it is done electronically or in print. This extends to creating a secondary or tertiary copy of the work or a recorded copy and is only allowed with the express written consent from the Publisher. All additional right reserved.

The information in the following pages is broadly considered a truthful and accurate account of facts and as such, any inattention, use, or misuse of the information in question by the reader will render any resulting actions solely under their purview. There are no scenarios in which the publisher or the original author of this work can be in any fashion deemed liable for any hardship or damages that may befall them after undertaking information described herein.

Additionally, the information in the following pages is intended only for informational purposes and should thus be thought of as universal. As befitting its nature, it is presented without assurance regarding its prolonged validity or interim quality. Trademarks that are mentioned are done without written consent and can in no way be considered an endorsement from the trademark holder.

WHAT IS DASH DIET ?

DASH stands for Dietary Approaches to Stop Hypertension. The DASH diet is a lifelong approach to healthy eating that's designed to help treat or prevent high blood pressure (hypertension).The DASH diet emphasizes vegetables, fruits and low-fat dairy foods and moderate amounts of whole grains, fish, poultry and nuts.

DASH may also affect other areas of health (Decreases cancer risk ,Lowers metabolic syndrome risk, Lowers diabetes risk, Decreases heart disease risk.)

The DASH Program :

Grains: 5 daily servings
Vegetables: 3 daily servings
Fruits: 4 daily servings
Low-fat or fat-free dairy products: 2 daily servings
Meat, poultry, and fish: 2 or less daily servings
So, you can pick and choose your favorite meals and enjoy them at any time of the day, from dawn to dusk.
You shouldn't expect DASH to help you shed weight on its own as it was designed fundamentally to lower blood pressure. Weight loss may simply be an added perk.

Look Inside

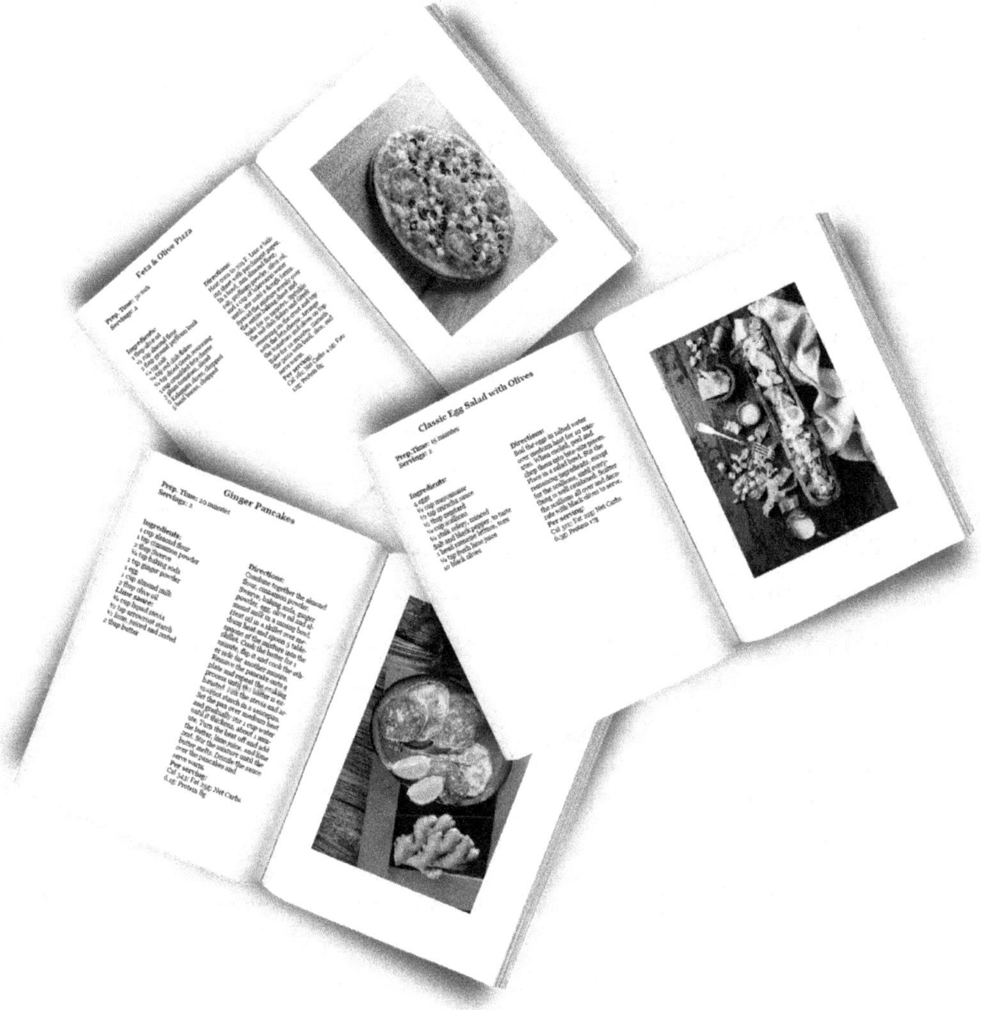

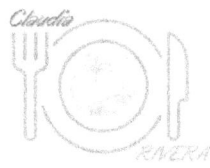

Table of Contents

Chapter 1 Breakfast — 8
Jalapeno Waffles with Bacon & Avocado — 9
Ginger Pancakes — 10
Belgium Waffles with Cheese Spread — 12
Spinach & Feta Cheese Pancakes — 14
Peanut Butter & Pastrami Gofres — 16

Chapter 2 Salads, Soups & Stews — 18
Kale & Broccoli Slaw with Bacon & Parmesan — 19
Classic Egg Salad with Olives — 20
Spinach & Brussels Sprout Salad — 22
Chicken Salad with Parmesan — 24
Smoked Mackerel Lettuce Cups — 26

Chapter 3 Vegetarian & Vegan — 28
Baked Veggies with Green Salad — 29
Roasted Pepper with Tofu — 30
Feta & Olive Pizza — 32
Chargrilled Zucchini with Avocado Pesto — 34
Walnut & Feta Loaf — 36

Chapter 4 Poultry & Meat — 38
Zucchini & Bell Pepper Chicken Gratin — 39
Paprika Chicken & Pancetta in a Skillet — 40
Green Bean & Broccoli Chicken Stir-Fry — 42
Roasted Pork Stuffed with Ham & Cheese — 44
Marinated Fried Chicken — 46

Chapter 5 Fish & Seafood — 48
Green Tuna Traybake — 49
Shirataki Fettucine with Salmon — 50
Tilapia Tortillas with Cauliflower Rice — 52
Chili Cod with Chive Sauce — 54
Grilled Tuna with Shirataki Pad Thai — 56

Chapter 6 Snacks, Appetizers & Side Dishes — 58
Camembert Bites with Blackberry Sauce — 59
Leafy Greens & Cheddar Quesadillas — 60

Cheese & Nut Zucchini Boats ------ 62
Baked Eggplant Chips with Salad & Aioli ------ 64
Mushroom & Cheese Lettuce Wraps ------ 66

Chapter 7 Desserts, Fruits & Drinks ------ 68
Mascarpone & Strawberry Pudding ------ 69
Minty Coconut Parfait with Cranberries ------ 70
Healthy Chia Pudding With Strawberries ------ 72
Chocolate Candies with Blueberries ------ 74
Matcha Brownies with Pistachios ------ 76

Chapter 8 Lunch ------ 78
Colorful Turkey Fajitas with Rotini Pasta ------ 79
Pasta Caprese with Ricotta & Basil ------ 80
Prep.Time: 15 minutes ------ 80
Soup Green Minestrone ------ 82
Sausage, Spinach & Tomato Rigatoni ------ 84
Spinach & Cheese Filled Conchiglie Shells ------ 86
Red Pepper & Chicken Fusilli ------ 88
Creamy Fettuccine with Ground Beef ------ 89

Chapter 9 Dinner ------ 91
Spinach, Garlic & Mushroom Pilaf ------ 92
Salmon & Tomato Farfalle ------ 94
Vegetarian Wild Rice with Carrots ------ 96
Risotto with Spring Vegetables & Shrimp ------ 98
Stuffed Mushrooms with Rice & Cheese ------ 100
Risotto with Broccoli & Grana Padano ------ 102
Arugula & Wild Mushroom Risotto ------ 104
Yummy Mexican-Style Rice & Pinto Beans ------ 106

Chapter 1 Breakfast

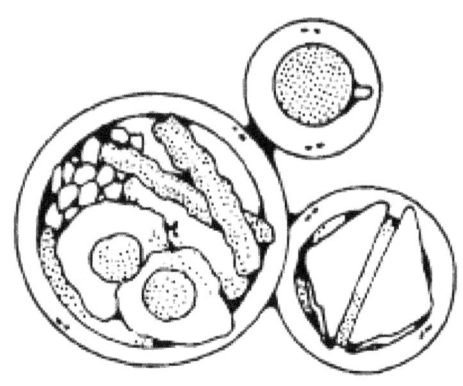

Jalapeno Waffles with Bacon & Avocado

Prep. Time: 20 minutes
Servings: 2

Ingredients:
2 tbsp butter, melted
¼ cup almond milk
2 tbsp almond flour
Salt and black pepper to taste
½ tsp parsley, chopped
½ jalapeño pepper, minced
4 eggs
½ cup cheddar, crumbled
4 slices bacon, chopped
1 avocado, sliced

Directions:
In a skillet over medium-low heat, fry the bacon until crispy, about 5 minutes. Remove to a plate. Combine the other ingredients in a bowl, except for the avocado. Preheat waffle iron and grease with cooking spray. After pouring the batter close the lid. Cook for 5 minutes or until the desired consistency is reached. Do the same with the rest of the batter. Top with avocado and bacon.

Per serving:
Cal 771; Fat 67g; Net Carbs 6.9g; Protein 27g

Ginger Pancakes

Prep. Time: 20 minutes
Servings: 2

Ingredients:
1 cup almond flour
1 tsp cinnamon powder
2 tbsp Swerve
¼ tsp baking soda
1 tsp ginger powder
1 egg
1 cup almond milk
2 tbsp olive oil

Lime sauce:
¼ cup liquid stevia
½ tsp arrowroot starch
½ lime, juiced and zested
2 tbsp butter

Directions:
Combine together the almond flour, cinnamon powder, Swerve, baking soda, ginger powder, egg, olive oil and almond milk in a mixing bowl. Heat oil in a skillet over medium heat and spoon 3 tablespoons of the mixture into the skillet. Cook the batter for 1 minute, flip it and cook the other side for another minute. Remove the pancake onto a plate and repeat the cooking process until the batter is exhausted. Mix the stevia and arrowroot starch in a saucepan. Set the pan over medium heat and gradually stir 1 cup water until it thickens, about 1 minute. Turn the heat off and add the butter, lime juice, and lime zest. Stir the mixture until the butter melts. Drizzle the sauce over the pancakes and serve warm.

Per serving:
Cal 343; Fat 25g; Net Carbs 6.1g; Protein 8g

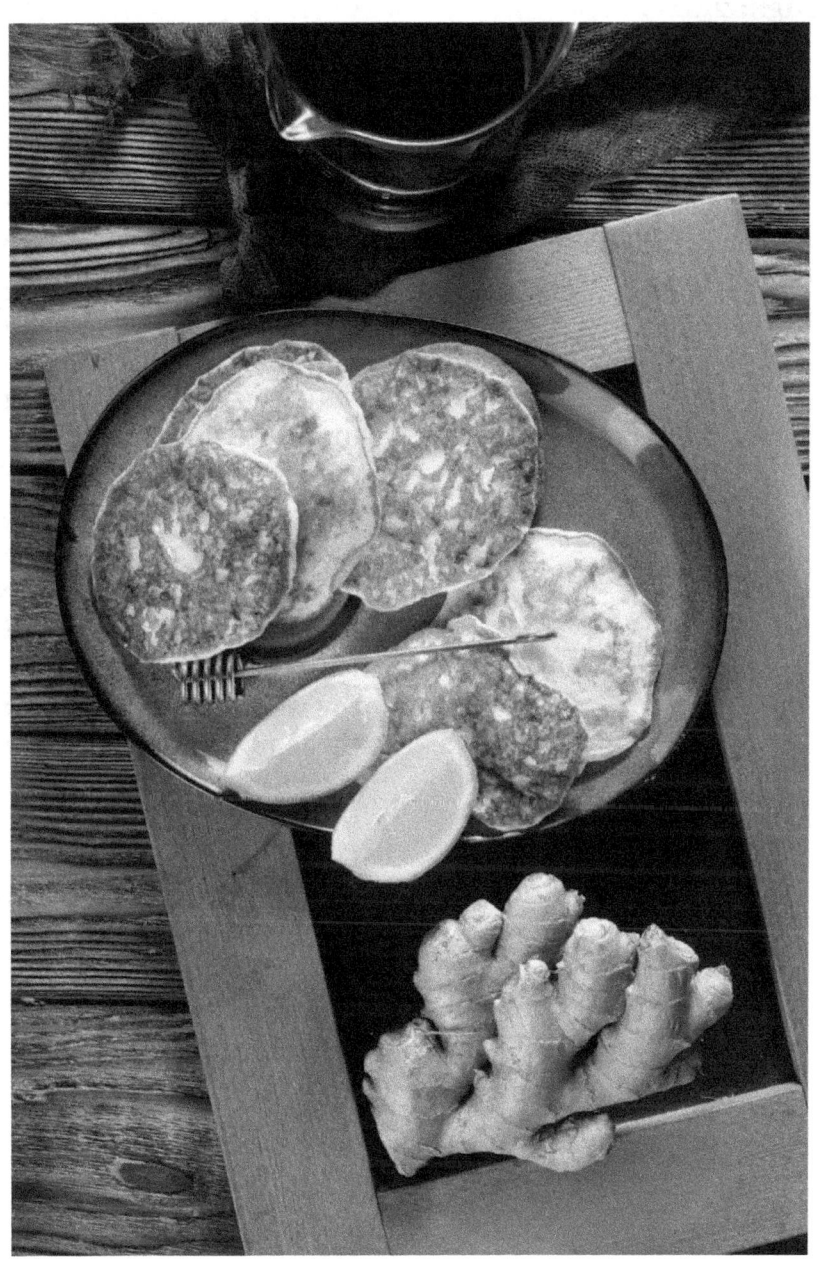

Belgium Waffles with Cheese Spread

Prep. Time: 25 minutes
Servings: 2

Ingredients:
½ cup cream cheese, softened
1 lemon, zested and juiced
2 tbsp liquid stevia
2 tbsp olive oil
½ cup almond milk
3 eggs
½ cup almond flour

Directions:
Combine, in a bowl, the cream cheese, lemon juice, lemon zest, and stevia. In a separate bowl, whisk the olive oil, almond milk, and eggs. Stir in almond flour and combine until no lumps exist. Let the batter sit for 5 minutes to thicken. Spritz a waffle iron with a cooking spray. Ladle a ¼ cup of the batter into the waffle iron and cook for about 5 minutes. Repeat with the remaining batter. Slice the waffles into quarters; apply the lemon spread in between each of two waffles, snap, and serve.

Per serving:
Cal 322; Fat 26g; Net Carbs 7.7g; Protein 11g

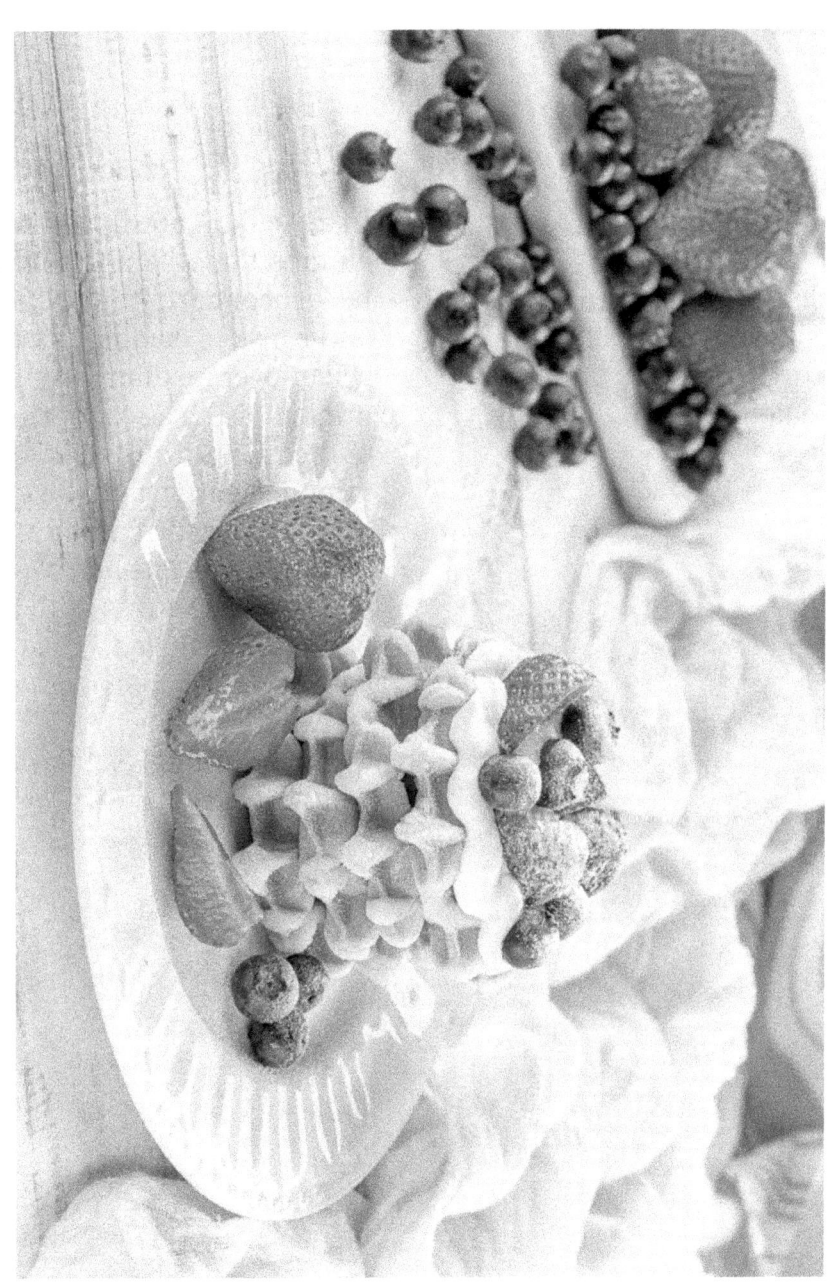

Spinach & Feta Cheese Pancakes

Prep. Time: 20 minutes
Servings: 2

Ingredients:
½ cup almond flour
½ tsp baking powder
½ cup feta cheese, crumbled
½ cup spinach, chopped
2 tbsp coconut milk
1 egg, beaten

Directions:
In a medium bowl, put the egg, almond flour, baking powder, feta, coconut milk, and spinach and whisk to combine. Set a skillet over medium heat for a minute. Fetch a soup spoonful of the mixture and cook for 2 minutes. Flip the pancake and cook further for 1 minute. Remove onto a plate and repeat the cooking process until the batter is exhausted. Serve with your favorite topping.

Per serving:
Cal 412; Fat 32g; Net Carbs 5.9g; Protein 12g

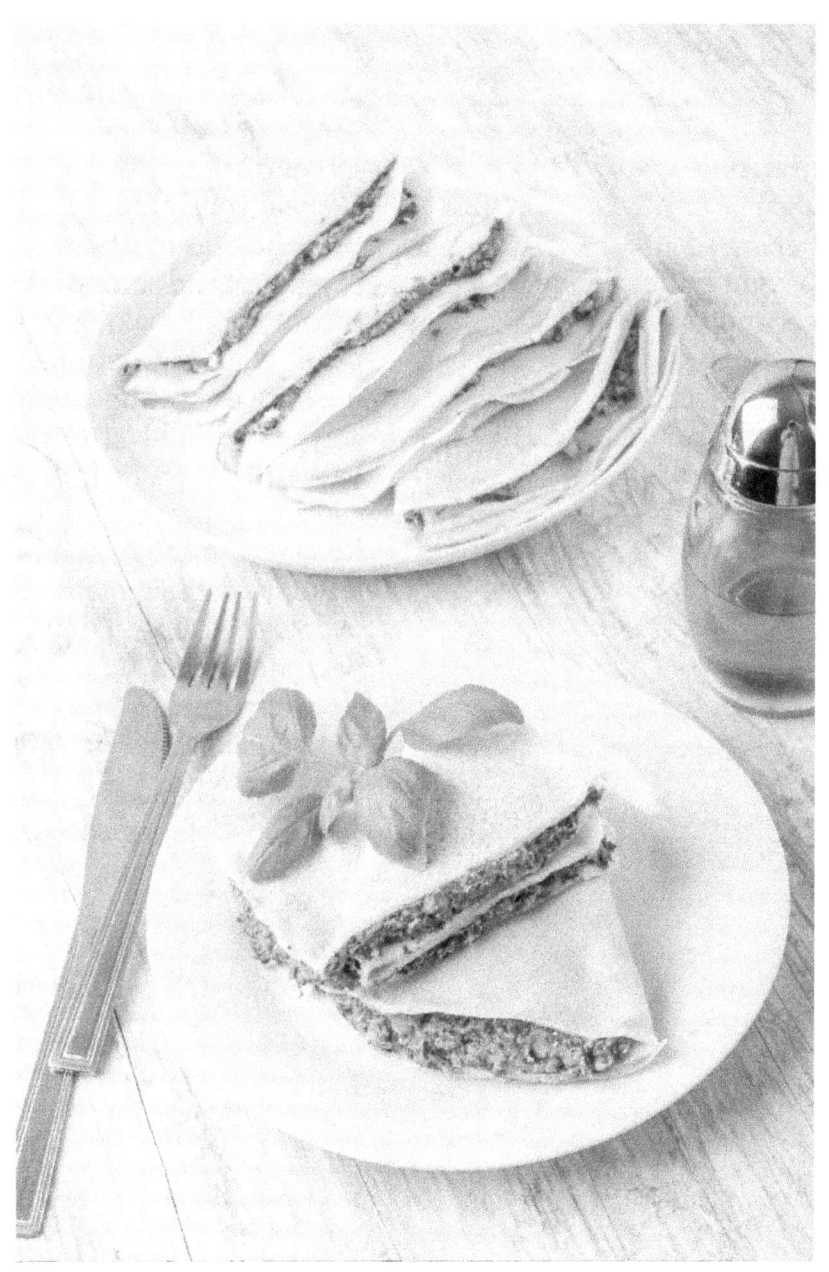

Peanut Butter & Pastrami Gofres

Prep. Time: 20 minutes
Servings: 2

Ingredients:
4 eggs
½ tsp baking soda
2 tbsp peanut butter, melted
4 tbsp coconut flour
¼ tsp salt
½ tsp dried rosemary
3 tbsp tomato puree
4 oz pastrami, chopped

Directions:
Preheat your waffle iron to high. Beat the eggs in a bowl with rosemary, and salt. Stir in the coconut flour, baking soda, and peanut butter. Continue whisking until everything is well incorporated. Add a third of the batter to the waffle iron and cook for 3 minutes until golden. Repeat with the remaining batter. Spread the tomato puree over each gofre and top with pastrami. Serve.

Per serving:
Cal 411; Fat 27g; Net Carbs 4.2g; Protein 25g

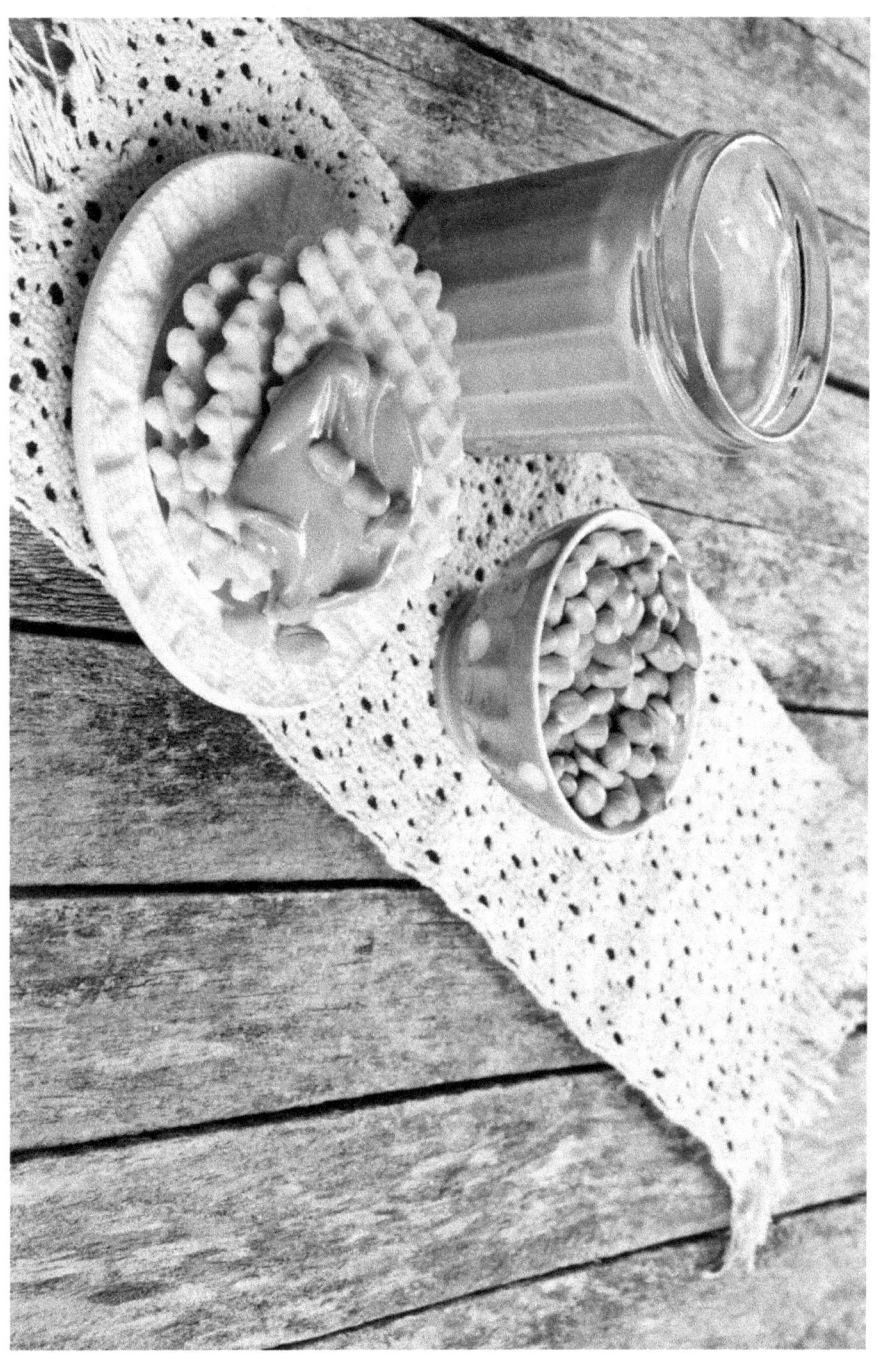

CHAPTER 2 SALADS, SOUPS & STEWS

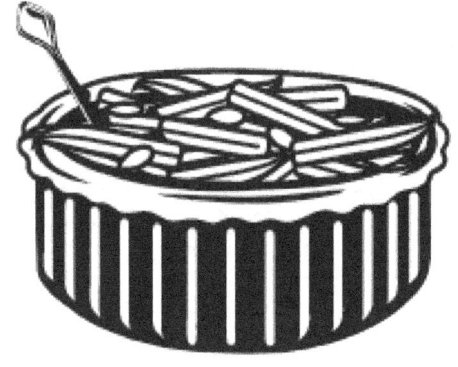

Kale & Broccoli Slaw with Bacon & Parmesan

Prep.Time: 10 minutes
Servings: 2

Ingredients:
2 tbsp olive oil
1 cup broccoli slaw
1 cup kale slaw
2 slices bacon, chopped
2 tbsp Parmesan, grated
1 tsp celery seeds
1 ½ tbsp apple cider vinegar
Salt and black pepper, to taste

Directions:
In a skillet fry the bacon over medium-high heat until crispy, about 5 minutes. Set aside to cool. In a salad bowl, whisk the vinegar, olive oil, salt, and pepper. Add in the broccoli, kale, and celery seeds and mix to combine well. Sprinkle with bacon and Parmesan and serve.

Per serving:
Cal 305; Fat 29g; Net Carbs 3.7g; Protein 7.3g

Classic Egg Salad with Olives

Prep.Time: 15 minutes
Servings: 2

Ingredients:
4 eggs
¼ cup mayonnaise
½ tsp sriracha sauce
½ tbsp mustard
¼ cup scallions
¼ stalk celery, minced
Salt and black pepper, to taste
1 head romaine lettuce, torn
¼ tsp fresh lime juice
10 black olives

Directions:
Boil the eggs in salted water over medium heat for 10 minutes. When cooled, peel and chop them into bite-size pieces. Place in a salad bowl. Stir the remaining ingredients, except for the scallions, until everything is well combined. Scatter the scallions all over and decorate with black olives to serve.

Per serving:
Cal 312; Fat 22g; Net Carbs 6.3g; Protein 17g

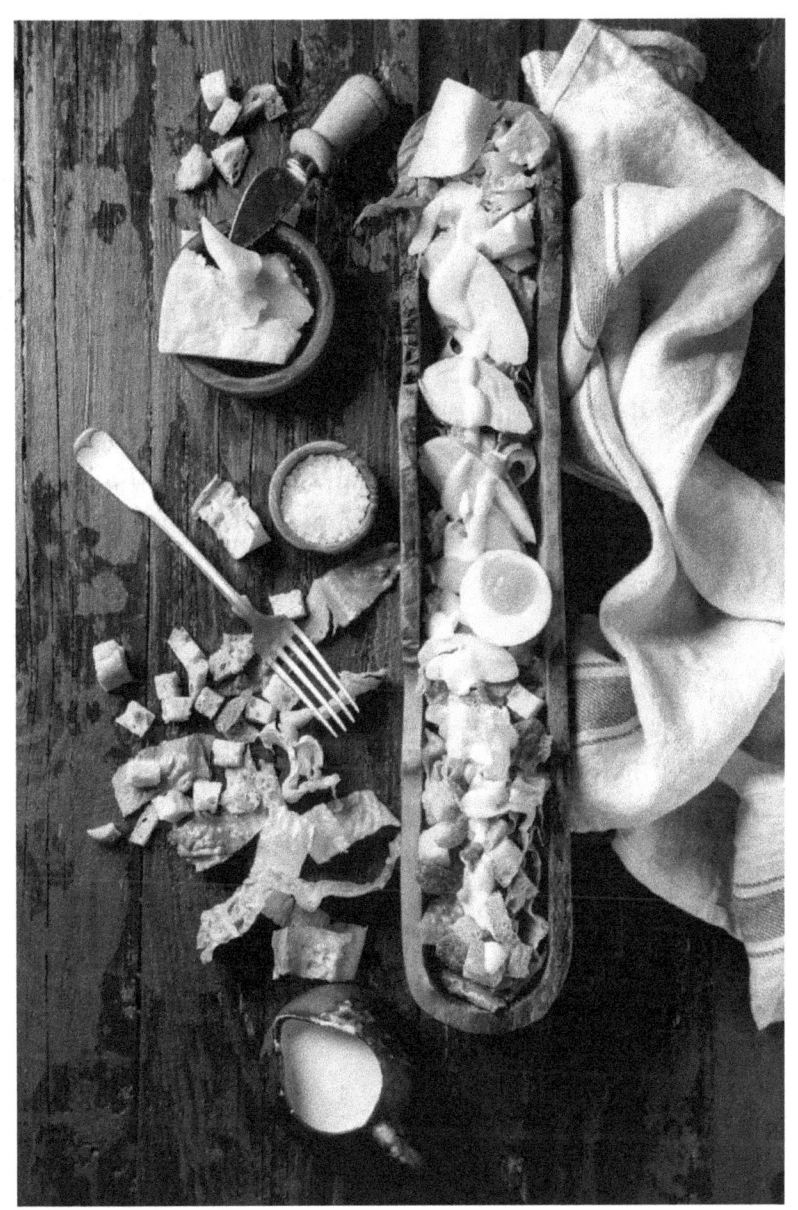

Spinach & Brussels Sprout Salad

Prep.Time: 35 minutes
Servings: 2

Ingredients:
1 lb Brussels sprouts, halved
2 tbsp olive oil
Salt and black pepper to taste
1 tbsp balsamic vinegar
2 tbsp extra virgin olive oil
1 cup baby spinach
1 tbsp Dijon mustard
½ cup hazelnuts

Directions:
Preheat oven to 400 F. Drizzle the Brussels sprouts with olive oil, sprinkle with salt and pepper, and spread on a baking sheet. Bake until tender, 20 minutes, tossing often. In a dry pan over medium-low heat, toast the hazelnuts for 2 minutes, cool, and then chop into small pieces. In a salad bowl put the brussels sprouts and add the baby spinach. Mix until well combined. In a bowl, combine vinegar, mustard, and olive oil. Drizzle the dressing over the salad and top with hazelnuts to serve.

Per serving:
Cal 511; Fat 43g; Net Carbs 9.6g; Protein 14g

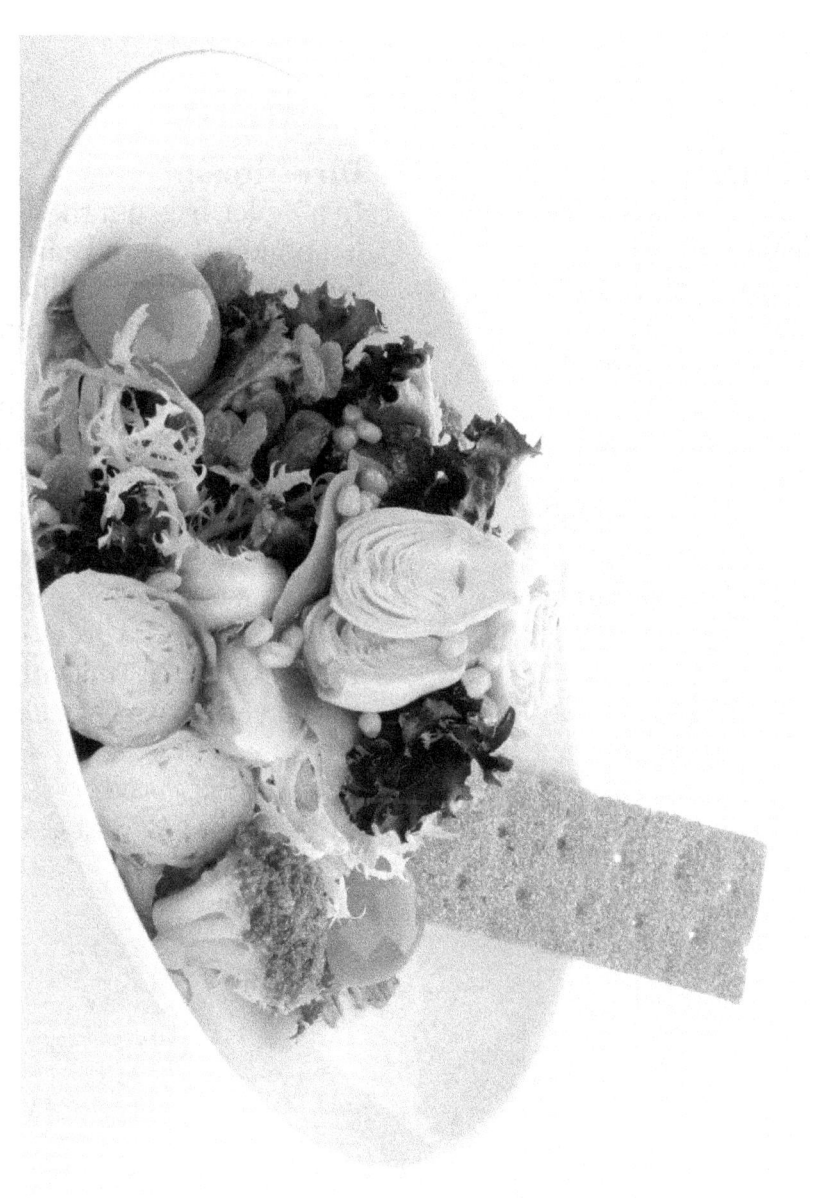

Chicken Salad with Parmesan

Prep.Time: 30 minutes
Servings: 2

Ingredients:
½ lb chicken breasts, sliced
¼ cup lemon juice
2 garlic cloves, minced
2 tbsp olive oil
1 romaine lettuce, shredded
3 Parmesan crisps
2 tbsp Parmesan, grated
Dressing:
2 tbsp extra virgin olive oil
1 tbsp lemon juice
Salt and black pepper to taste

Directions:
In a Ziploc bag, put the chicken, lemon juice, oil, and garlic. Seal the bag, shake to combine, and refrigerate for 1 hour. Preheat the grill to medium-low heat and grill the chicken for about 2-3 minutes per side. Combine the dressing ingredients in a medium-large bowl and mix well. On a serving platter, arrange the lettuce and Parmesan crisps. Scatter the dressing over and toss to coat. Top with the chicken and Parmesan cheese to serve.

Per serving:
Cal 529; Fat 36g; Net Carbs 4.3g; Protein 34g

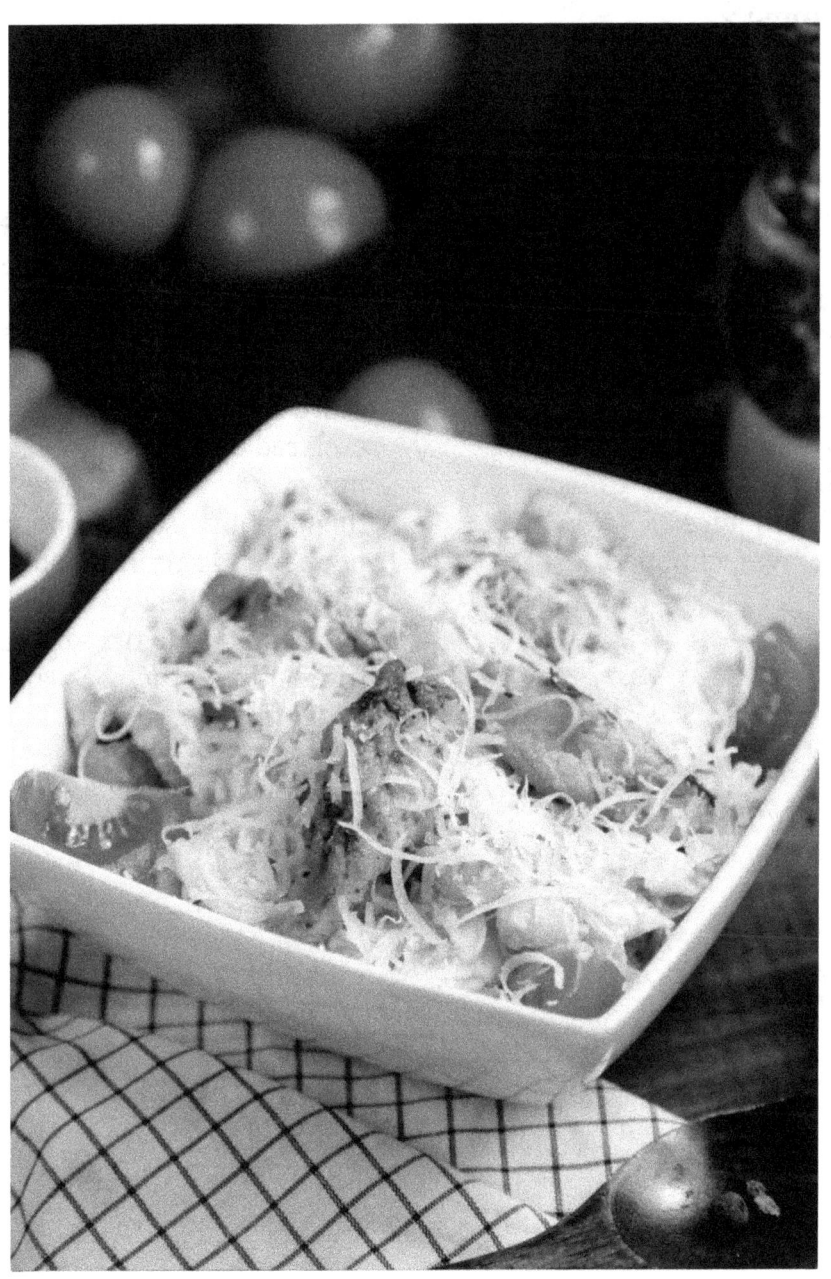

Smoked Mackerel Lettuce Cups

Prep.Time: 20 minutes
Servings: 2

Ingredients:
½ head Iceberg lettuce, firm leaves removed for cups
4 oz smoked mackerel, flaked
Salt and black pepper to taste
2 eggs
1 tomato, seeded, chopped
2 tbsp mayonnaise
¼ red onion, sliced
1 tsp lemon juice
1 tbsp chives, chopped

Directions:
In a small pot boil the eggs with salted water for 10 minutes. Then, run the eggs in cold water, peel, and chop into small pieces. Transfer them to a salad bowl. Add in the smoked mackerel, red onion, and tomato and mix evenly with a spoon. Mix the mayonnaise, lemon juice, pepper and salt in a small bowl. Lay two lettuce leaves each as cups and divide the salad mixture between them. Sprinkle with chives and serve.

Per serving:
Cal 314; Fat 25g; Net Carbs 3g; Protein 16g

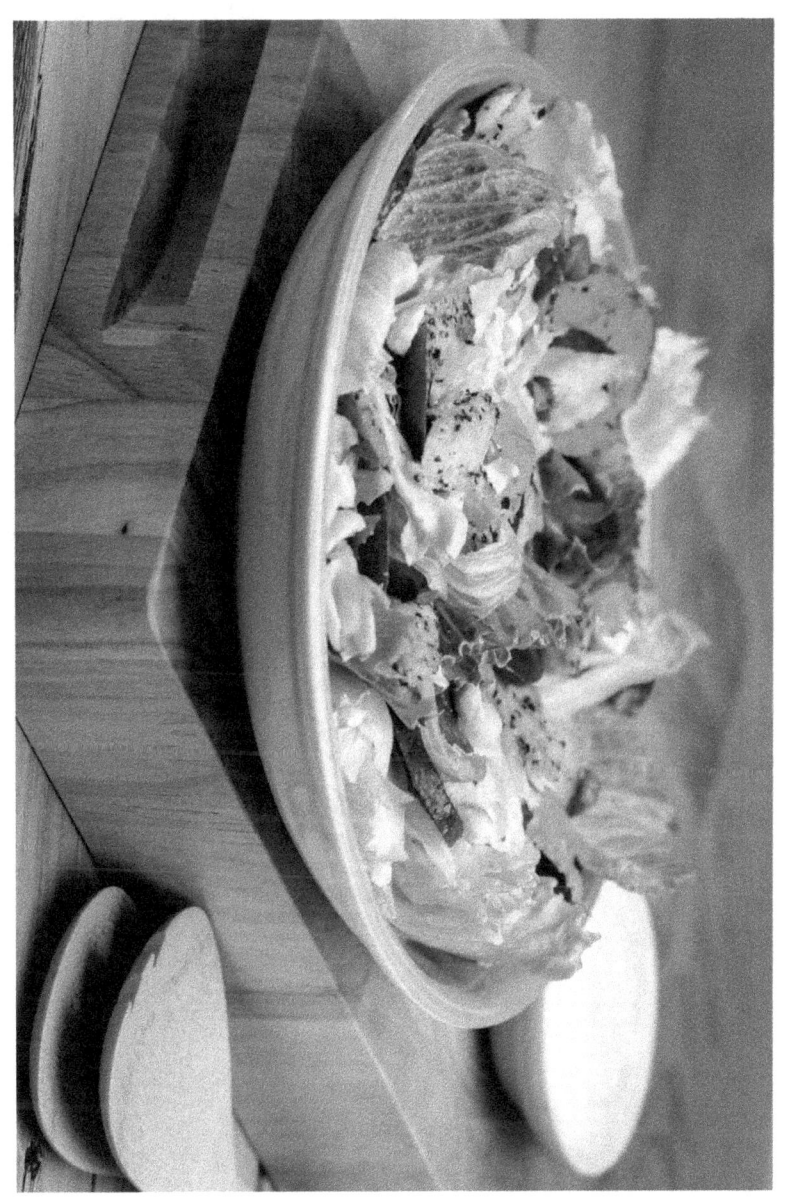

CHAPTER 3 VEGETARIAN & VEGAN

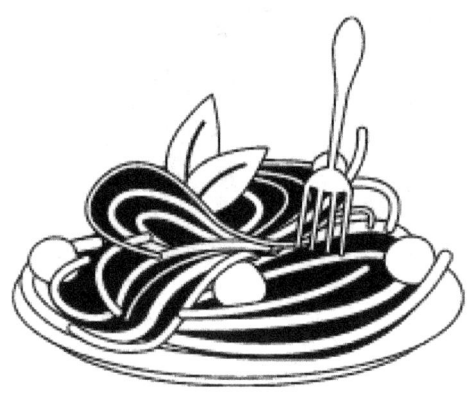

Baked Veggies with Green Salad

Prep. Time: 30 min
Servings: 2

Ingredients:
1 zucchini, sliced
1 eggplant, sliced
¼ cup coconut oil
2 tbsp pecans
Juice of ½ lemon
5 oz cheddar cheese, cubed
10 Kalamata olives
1 oz mixed salad greens
½ cup mayonnaise
½ tsp Cayenne pepper

Directions;
Line a baking sheet with parchment paper. Arrange zucchini and eggplant slices on the sheet. Brush with coconut oil and sprinkle with cayenne pepper. Setting the oven to broil, bake the vegetables until golden brown, about 18-20 minutes. Remove to a serving platter and drizzle with lemon juice. Arrange cheddar cheese, olives, pecans, and mixed greens next to baked veggies. Top with mayonnaise and serve.

Per serving:
Cal 509g; Net Carbs 8g; Fat 31g; Protein 22g

Roasted Pepper with Tofu

Prep. Time: 25 min
Servings: 4

Ingredients:
2 ½ cups cubed tofu
4 orange bell peppers
1 cucumber, diced
1 large tomato, chopped
3 oz cream cheese
¾ cup mayonnaise
1 tbsp melted butter
1 tsp dried parsley
1 tsp dried basil
Salt and black pepper to taste

Directions:
Preheat a broiler to 450 F. Line a baking sheet with parchment paper. In a salad bowl, combine cream cheese, mayonnaise, cucumber, tomato, salt, pepper, and parsley; refrigerate. Arrange bell peppers and tofu on the baking sheet, drizzle with melted butter, and season with basil, salt, and pepper. Bake for 15-17 minutes until the peppers have charred lightly and the tofu browned. Serve with chilled salad and enjoy!
Per serving: Cal 838; Net Carbs 8g; Fat 81g; Protein 31g

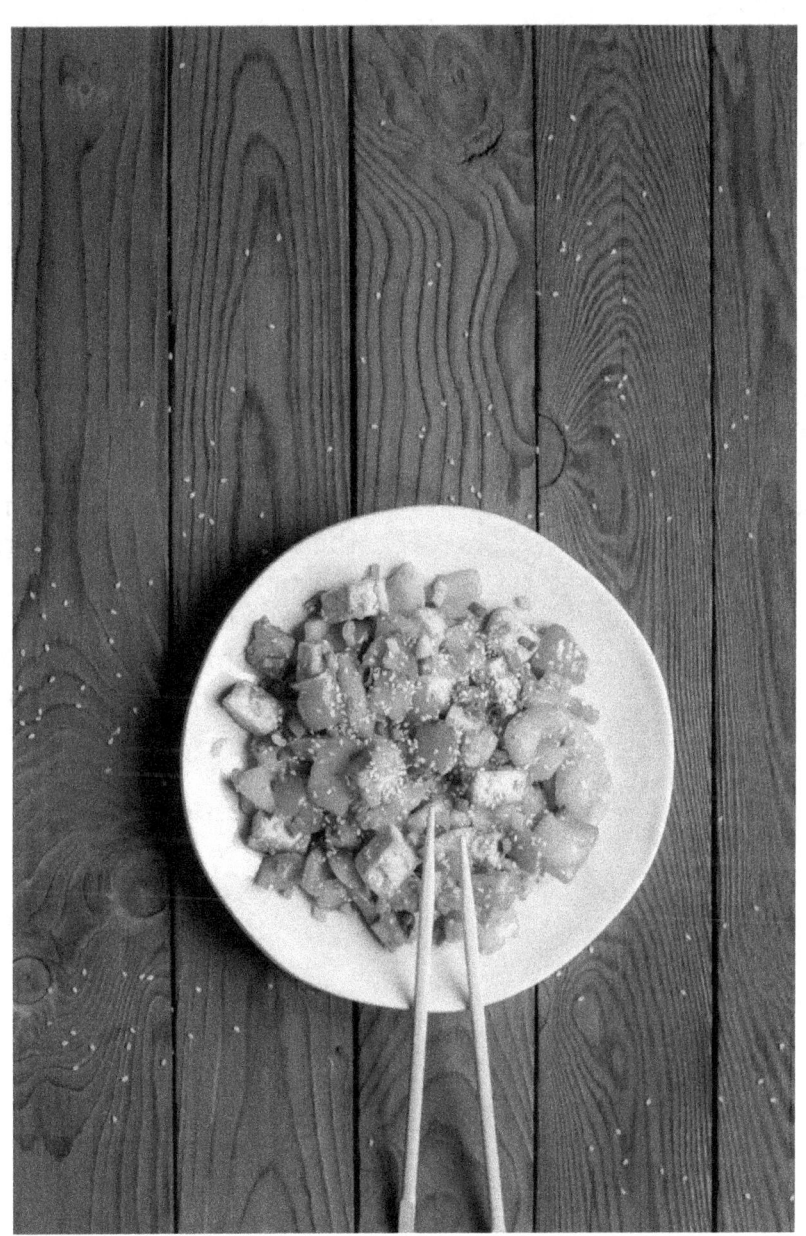

Feta & Olive Pizza

Prep. Time: 30 min
Servings: 4

Ingredients:
1 tbsp olive oil
½ cup almond flour
2 tbsp ground psyllium husk
¼ tsp salt
¼ tsp red chili flakes
¼ tsp dried Greek seasoning
1 cup crumbled feta cheese
3 plum tomatoes, sliced
6 Kalamata olives, chopped
5 basil leaves, chopped

Directions:
Heat oven to 395 F. Line a baking sheet with parchment paper. In a bowl, mix almond flour, salt, psyllium powder, olive oil, and 1 cup of lukewarm water until; stir until a dough forms. Spread the mixture evenly over the entire baking sheet and bake for 10 minutes. Sprinkle the red chili flakes and Greek seasoning on the crust and top with the feta cheese. Arrange the tomatoes and olives on top. Bake for 10 minutes. Garnish the pizza with basil, slice, and serve warm.

Per serving:
Cal 281; Net Carbs 4.5g; Fats 12g; Protein 8g

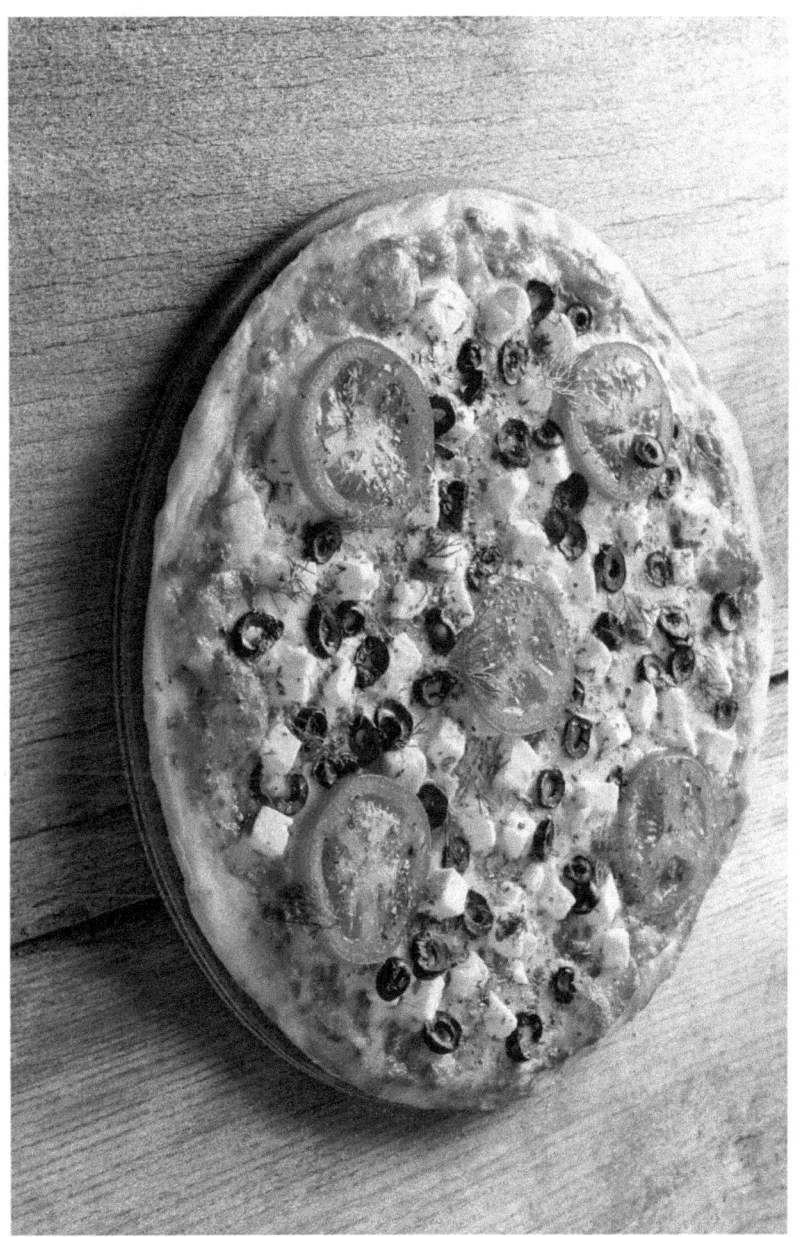

Chargrilled Zucchini with Avocado Pesto

Prep. Time: 20 min
Servings: 4

Ingredients:
1 avocado, chopped
3 oz spinach, chopped
2 zucchinis, sliced
¾ cup olive oil
2 tbsp melted butter
2 oz pecans
1 garlic clove, minced
Juice of 1 lemon
Salt and black pepper to taste

Directions:
Transfer the spinach in a food processor and avocado, lemon juice, garlic, olive oil, and pecans and blend until smooth and fluid; then season with salt and black pepper. Pour the pesto into a medium bowl and set it aside. Season zucchini with salt, pepper, and butter. Preheat a grill pan over medium-low heat and cook the zucchini slices until browned, 8-10 minutes in total. Remove to a plate, spoon the pesto to the side, and serve.

Per serving:
Cal 548; Net Carbs 6g; Fat 46g; Protein 25g

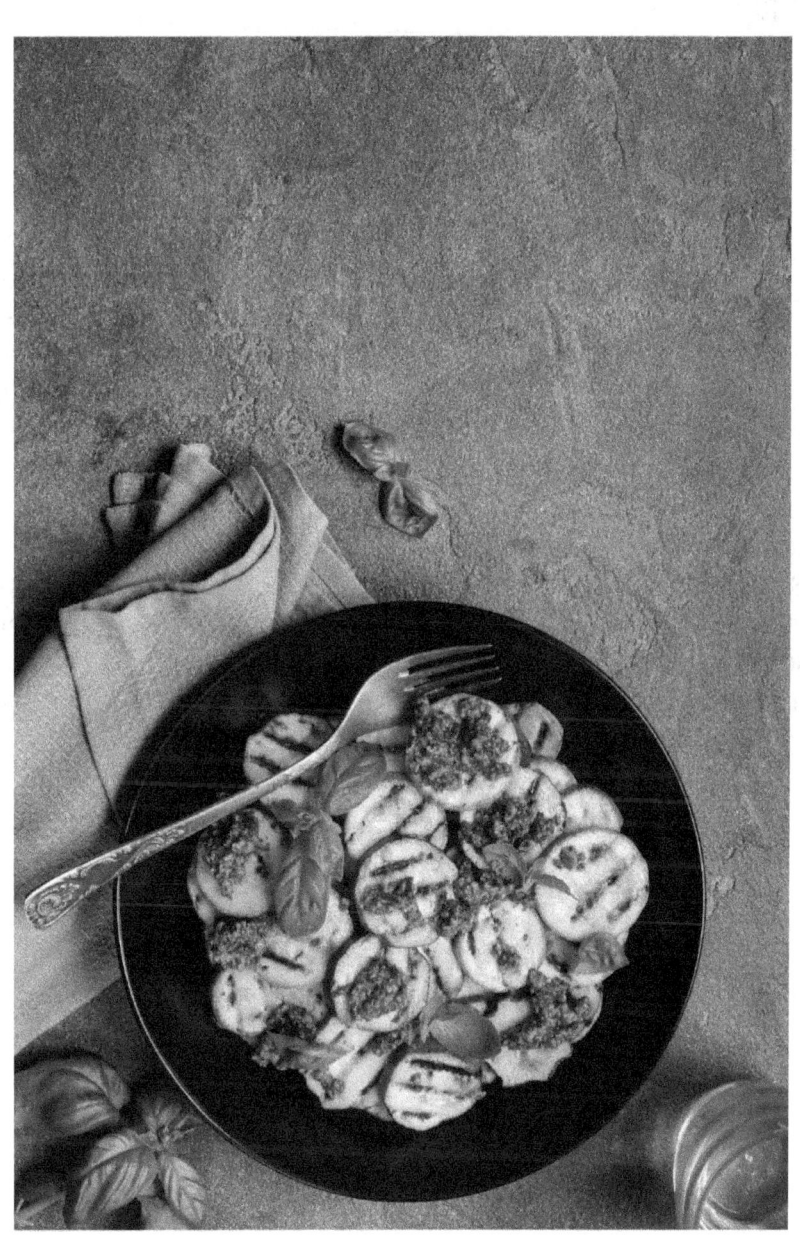

Walnut & Feta Loaf

Prep. Time: 60 min
Servings: 4

Ingredients:
1 green bell pepper, chopped
1 red bell pepper, chopped
2 white onions, chopped
4 garlic cloves, minced
1 lb feta, cubed
3 tbsp olive oil
2 tbsp soy sauce
¾ cup chopped walnuts
Salt and black pepper
1 tbsp Italian mixed herbs
½ tsp Swerve sugar
¼ cup golden flaxseed meal
1 tbsp sesame seeds
½ cup tomato sauce

Directions:
Preheat oven to 350 F. In a bowl, combine olive oil, onions, garlic, feta, soy sauce, walnuts, salt, pepper, Italian herbs, Swerve, and flaxseed meal and mix with your hands. Pour and mix the mixture in a bowl with the sesame seeds and peppers. Transfer the mixture into a greased loaf and spoon tomato sauce on top. Bake for 45 minutes. Turn onto a chopping board, slice, and serve.

Per serving: Cal 429; Net Carbs 2.5g; Fat 28g; Protein 24g

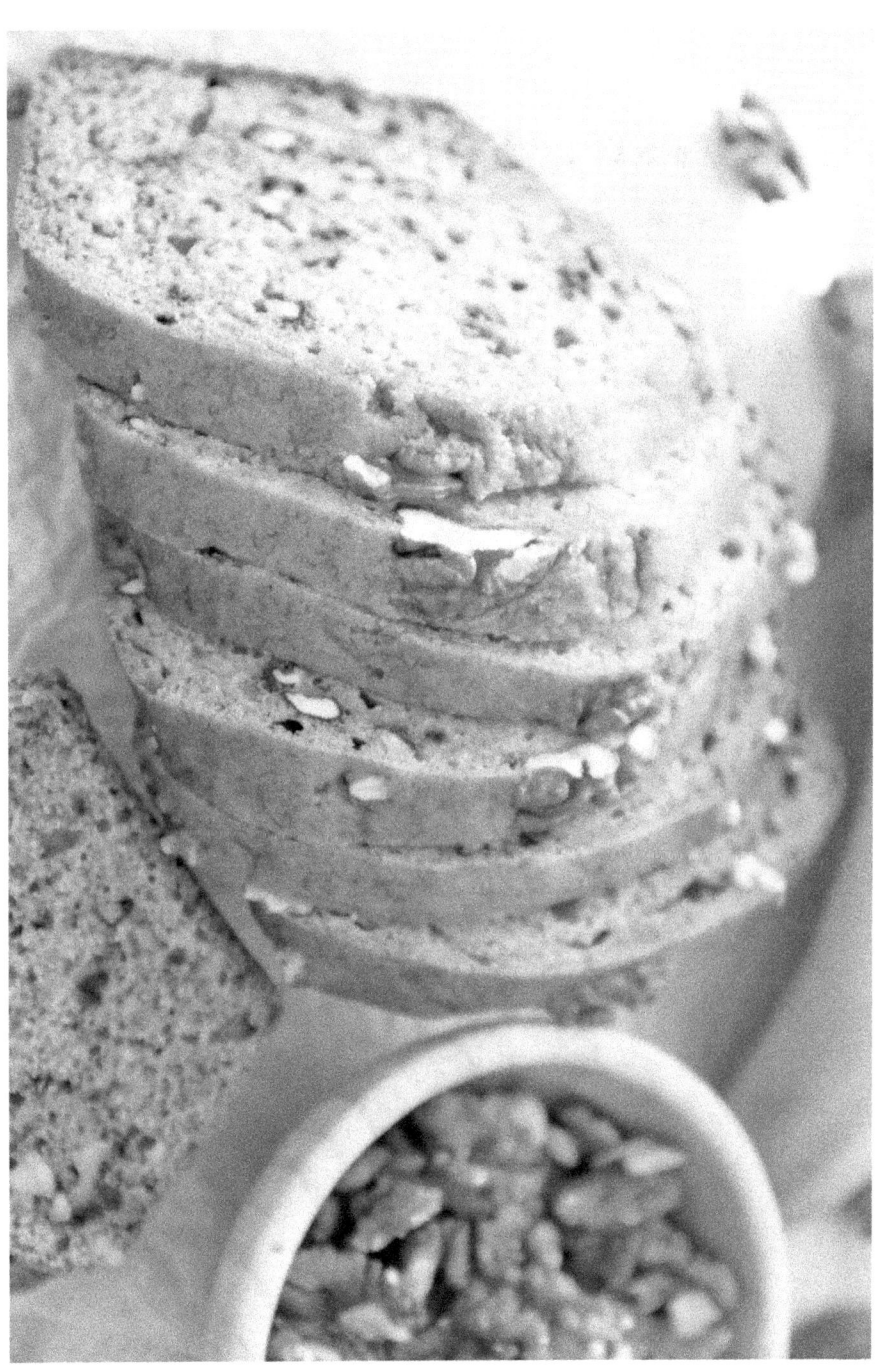

Chapter 4 Poultry & Meat

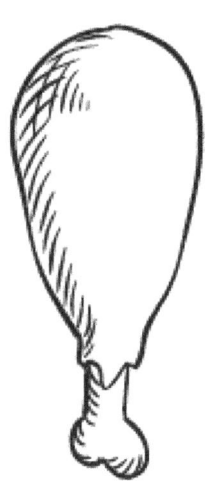

Zucchini & Bell Pepper Chicken Gratin

Prep.Time: 40 minutes
Servings: 2

Ingredients:
1 red bell pepper, sliced
1 zucchini, chopped
Salt and black pepper, to taste
1 tsp garlic powder
1 tbsp olive oil
2 chicken breasts, sliced
1 tomato, chopped
½ tsp dried oregano
½ tsp dried basil
½ cup mozzarella, shredded

Directions:
Coat the chicken with salt, black pepper and garlic powder. Warm olive oil in a skillet over medium heat and add in the chicken slices. Cook until golden and remove to a baking dish. To the same pan, add the zucchini, tomato, bell pepper, basil, oregano, and salt and cook for 2 minutes. Spread the mixture over the chicken. Bake at 370 F for 18-20 minutes in the oven. Sprinkle the mozzarella over the chicken, return to the oven, and bake for 5 minutes until the cheese is melted and bubbling. Serve.

Per serving:
Cal 467; Fat 23g; Net Carbs 6.2g; Protein 45g

Paprika Chicken & Pancetta in a Skillet

Prep.Time: 35 minutes
Servings: 2

Ingredients:
1 tbsp olive oil
5 pancetta strips, chopped
1/3 cup Dijon mustard
Salt and black pepper to taste
1 onion, chopped
1 cup chicken stock
2 chicken breasts
¼ tsp sweet paprika
2 tbsp oregano, chopped

Directions:
In a bowl, combine the paprika, black pepper, salt, and mustard. Rub the mixture onto the chicken breasts. In a skillet, place the oil and heat it over medium heat. Add the pancetta and cook for about 3-4 minutes; remove to a plate. To the pancetta fat, add the chicken breasts and cook for 2 minutes per side. Place in the stock, black pepper, pancetta, salt, and onion. Simmer for 15-20 minutes. Sprinkle with oregano and serve.

Per serving:
Cal 323; Fat 21g; Net Carbs 4.6g; Protein 24g

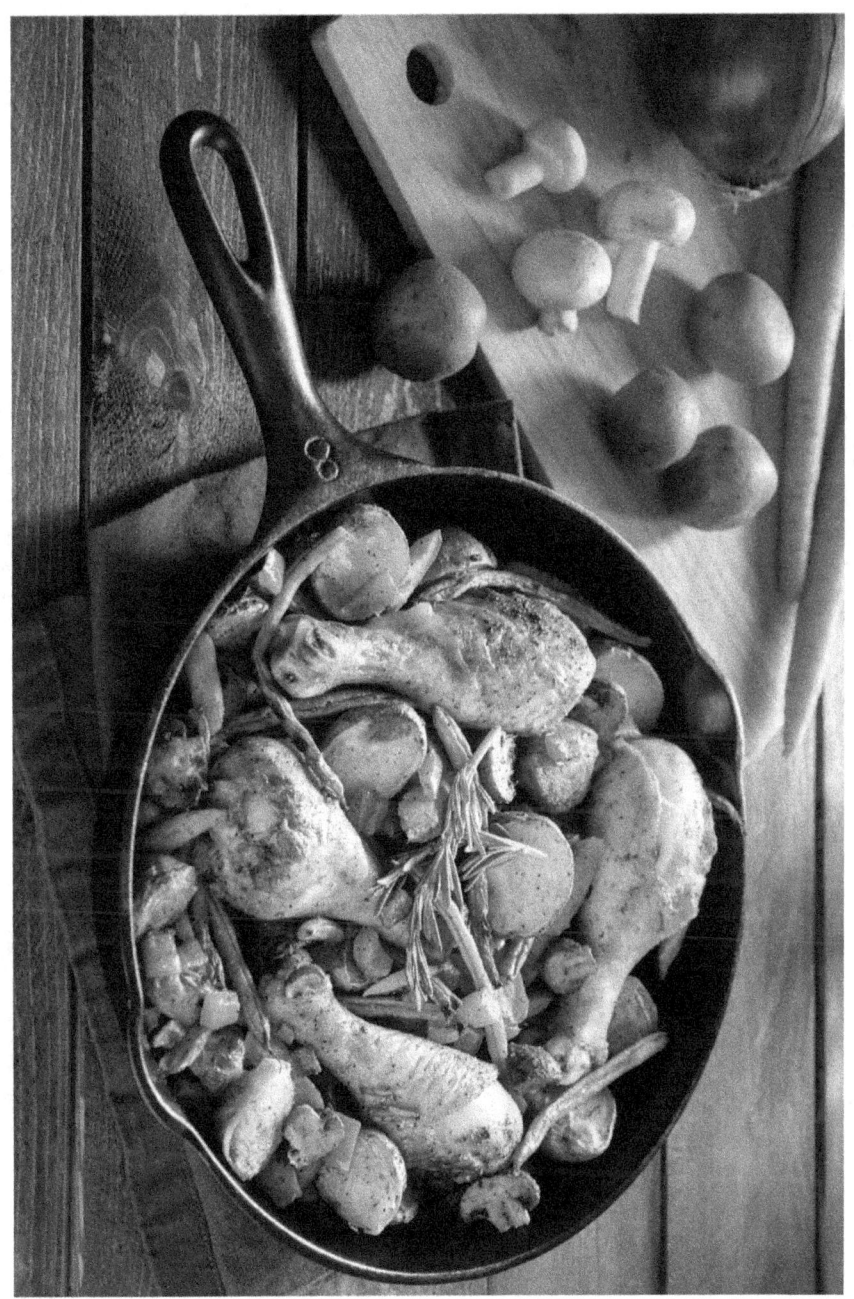

Green Bean & Broccoli Chicken Stir-Fry

Prep.Time: 45 minutes
Servings: 2

Ingredients:
2 chicken breasts, cut into strips
2 tbsp olive oil
1 tsp red pepper flakes
1 tsp onion powder
1 tbsp fresh ginger, grated
¼ cup tamari sauce
½ tsp garlic powder
½ cup water
½ cup xylitol
4 oz green beans, chopped
½ tsp xanthan gum
½ cup green onions, chopped
10 oz broccoli florets

Directions:
Steam the green beans and broccoli for 5-6 minutes until it is crisp-tender but still vibrant green; set aside.
Warm the olive oil in a pan over medium heat and cook the chicken and ginger for 4 minutes. Mix in the remaining ingredients and bake for 15 minutes. Return the green beans and broccoli and cook for 6 minutes. Serve.

Per serving:
Cal 411; Fat 25g; Net Carbs 6.2g; Protein 28g

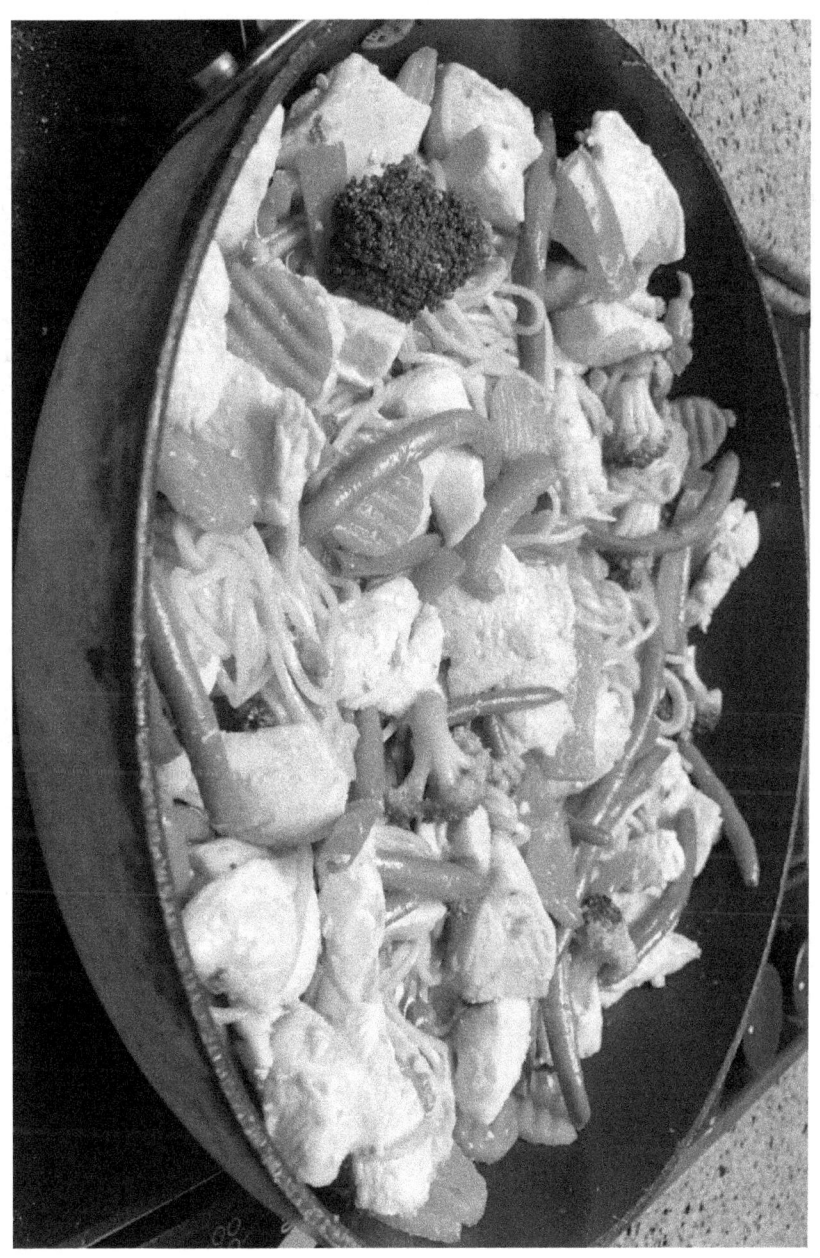

Roasted Pork Stuffed with Ham & Cheese

Prep.Time: 40 minutes
Servings: 2

Ingredients:
2 tbsp olive oil
Zest and juice from 1 lime
1 garlic clove, minced
2 tbsp fresh cilantro, chopped
2 tbsp fresh mint, chopped
Salt and black pepper to taste
1 tsp cumin
2 pork loin steaks
1 pickle, chopped
2 oz smoked ham, sliced
2 oz Gruyere cheese sliced
1 tbsp mustard

Directions:
Combine the lime zest, oil, black pepper, cumin, cilantro, lime juice, garlic, mint, and salt in a food processor; transfer to a bowl. Place the steaks in the marinade and toss well to coat. Place in the fridge for 2 hours. Preheat oven to 360 F. Arrange the steaks on a working surface, split the pickles, mustard, cheese, and ham on them, roll, and secure with toothpicks. Heat a pan over medium-low heat, add in the pork rolls, cook each side for 2 minutes and remove to a baking sheet. Bake in the oven at 350 F for 25 minutes. Serve and enjoy!

Per serving:
Cal 433; Fat 38g; Net Carbs 4.2g; Protein 24g

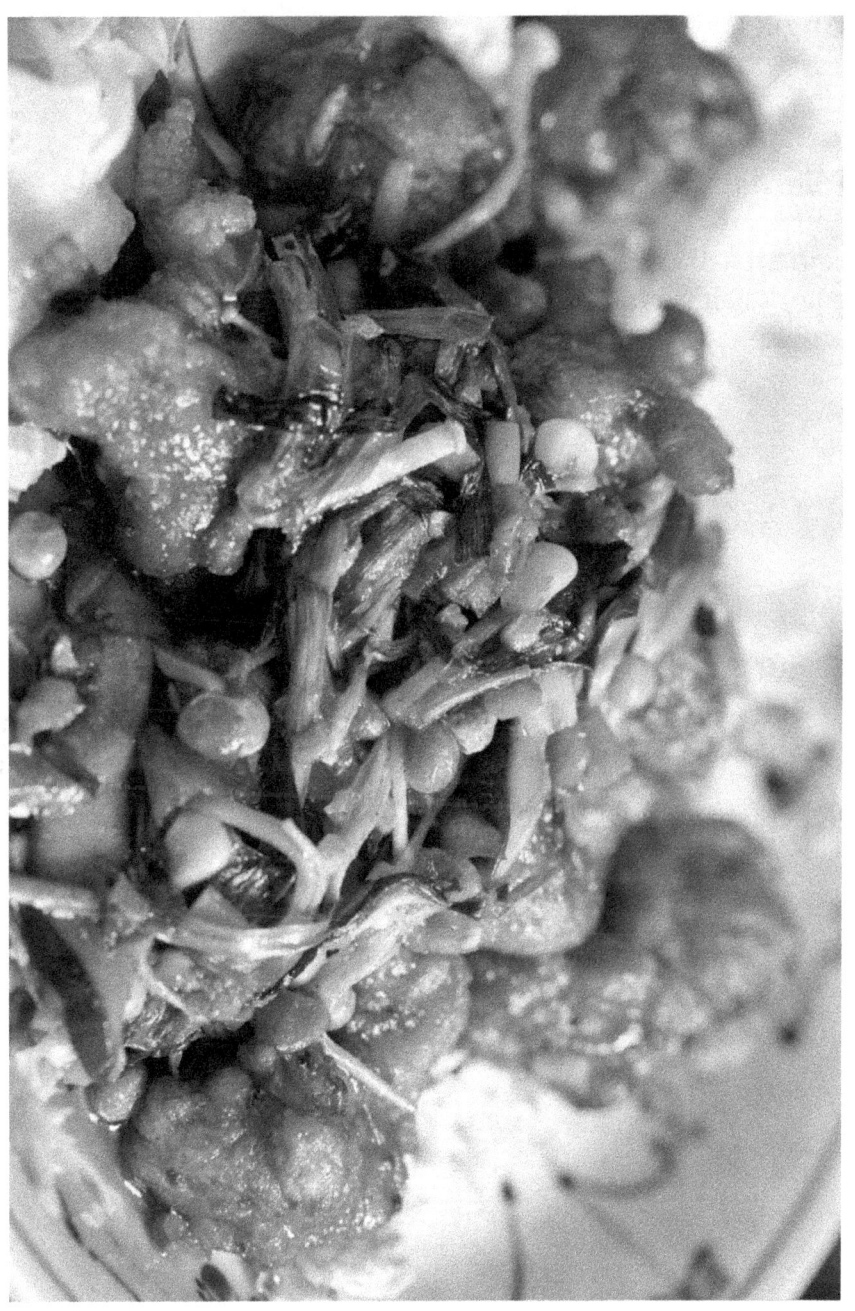

Marinated Fried Chicken

Prep.Time: 15 minutes
Servings: 2

Ingredients:
2 tbsp olive oil
2 chicken breasts, cut into strips
½ cup pork rinds, crushed
8 oz jarred pickle juice
1 egg

Directions:
Cover the chicken with pickle juice in a bowl and refrigerate for 12 hours while covered. Whisk the egg in a bowl, and place the pork rinds in a separate bowl. Dip the chicken pieces in the egg, then in the pork rinds. Ensure they are well coated. Place the oil in a medium skillet and heat over medium heat. Fry the chicken for 3 minutes on each side, remove to paper towels, and drain the excess grease. Serve warm with homemade ketchup if desired.

Per serving:
Cal 393; Fat 16g; Net Carbs 3.1g; Protein 21g

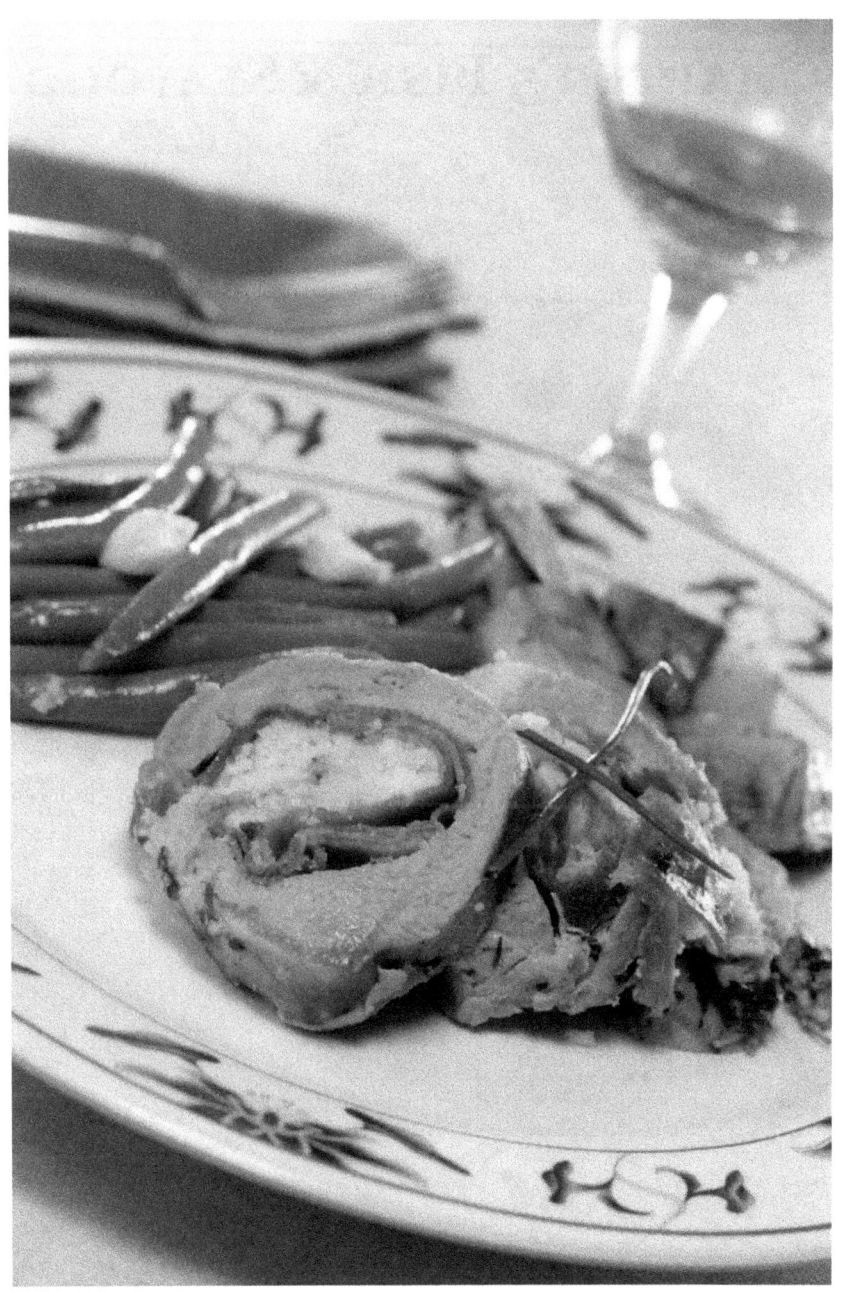

CHAPTER 5 FISH & SEAFOOD

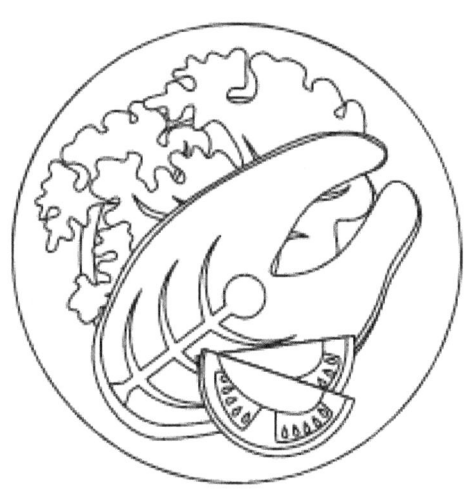

Green Tuna Traybake

Prep. Time: 45 min
Servings: 4

Ingredients:
1 (15 oz) can tuna in water, drained and flaked
1 bunch asparagus, trimmed and cut into 1-inch pieces
1 cup green beans, chopped
1 tbsp butter
2 tbsp arrowroot starch
2 cups coconut milk
4 zucchinis, spiralized
1 cup grated Parmesan cheese

Directions:
Preheat the oven to 370 F. Melt butter in a skillet and sauté the green beans and asparagus until softened, about 5 minutes; set aside. In a saucepan over medium heat, mix arrowroot starch with coconut milk. Bring to a boil and cook with frequent stirring until thickened, 3 minutes. Stir in half of Parmesan cheese until melted. Mix in the green beans, asparagus, zucchinis, and tuna. Transfer the mixture to a baking dish and sprinkle with the remaining Parmesan cheese. Bake until the cheese is melted and golden, 18-20 minutes. Serve.

Per serving:
Cal 392; Net Carbs 8g; Fats 34g; Protein 9g

Shirataki Fettucine with Salmon

Prep. Time: 35 min
Servings: 4

Ingredients:
4 salmon fillets, cubed
8 oz shirataki fettuccine
5 tbsp butter
3 garlic cloves, minced
1 ¼ cups heavy cream
½ cup dry white wine
1 tsp lemon zest
1 cup baby spinach
Salt and black pepper to taste

Directions:
Pour 2,5 cups of water into a pot and bring it to a boil. Strain the shirataki pasta and rinse well under hot running water. Allow proper draining and pour the shirataki pasta into the boiling water. Cook for 3 minutes and strain again. Place in a dry skillet over medium heat and stir-fry the shirataki pasta until visibly dry, 1-2 minutes; set aside. Cook half of the butter in the skillet. Season the salmon with salt and pepper and cook for 8 minutes, stirring occasionally; set aside. Melt the remaining butter in the skillet and stir-fry the garlic for 30 seconds. Mix in heavy cream, wine, lemon zest, salt, and pepper. Cook over low heat for 5 minutes. Stir in spinach, let wilt for 2 minutes. Stir in shirataki fettuccine and salmon. Serve.

Per serving:
Cal 803; Net Carbs 9g; Fats 46g; Protein 69g

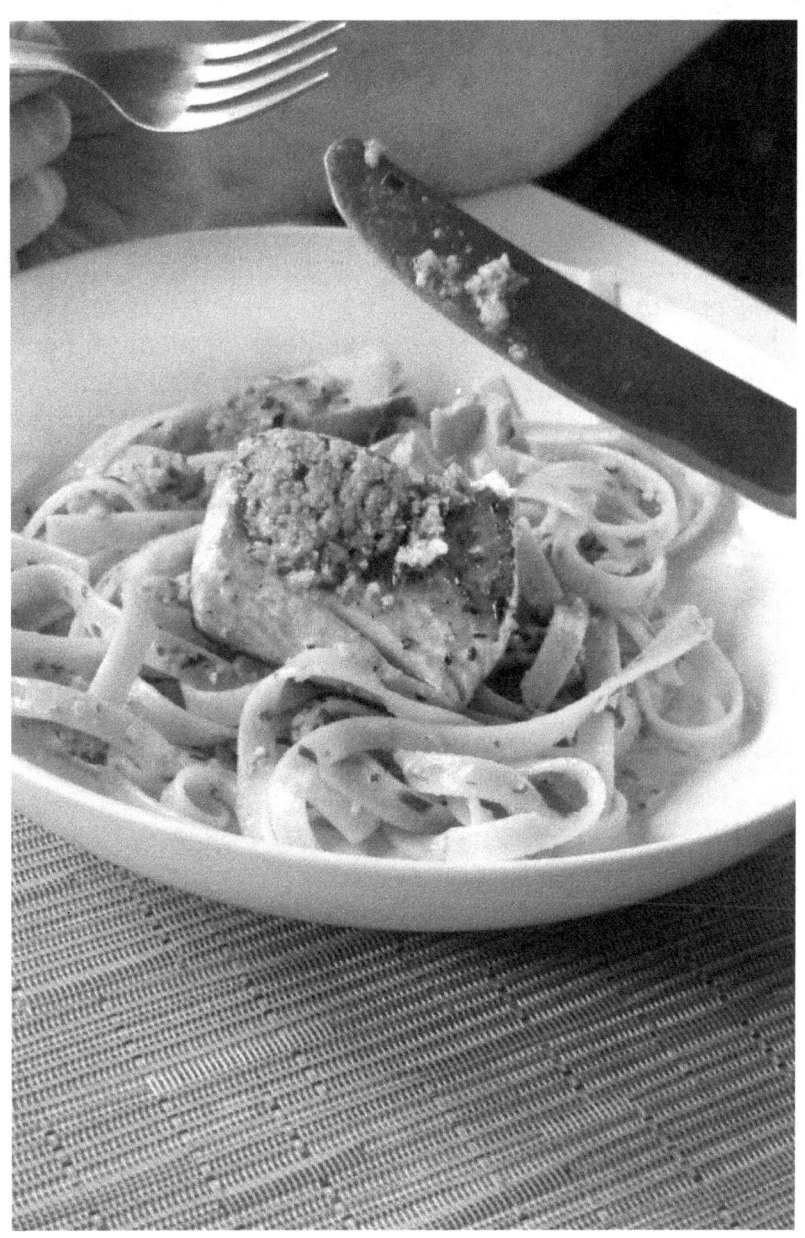

Tilapia Tortillas with Cauliflower Rice

Prep. Time: 20 min
Servings: 2

Ingredients:
1 tsp avocado oil
1 cup cauli rice
2 tilapia fillets, cut into cubes
¼ tsp taco seasoning
Salt and hot paprika to taste
2 whole cabbage leaves
2 tbsp guacamole
1 tbsp cilantro, chopped

Directions:
Microwave the cauli rice in a microwave-safe bowl for 4 minutes. Fluff with a fork and set aside. Warm avocado oil in a skillet over medium heat, rub the tilapia with the taco seasoning, salt, and hot paprika and fry until brown on all sides, about 8 minutes in total.
Divide the fish among the cabbage leaves, top with cauli rice, guacamole, and cilantro. Serve.

Per serving:
Cal 170; Fat 6.4g; Net Carbs 1.4g; Protein 24g

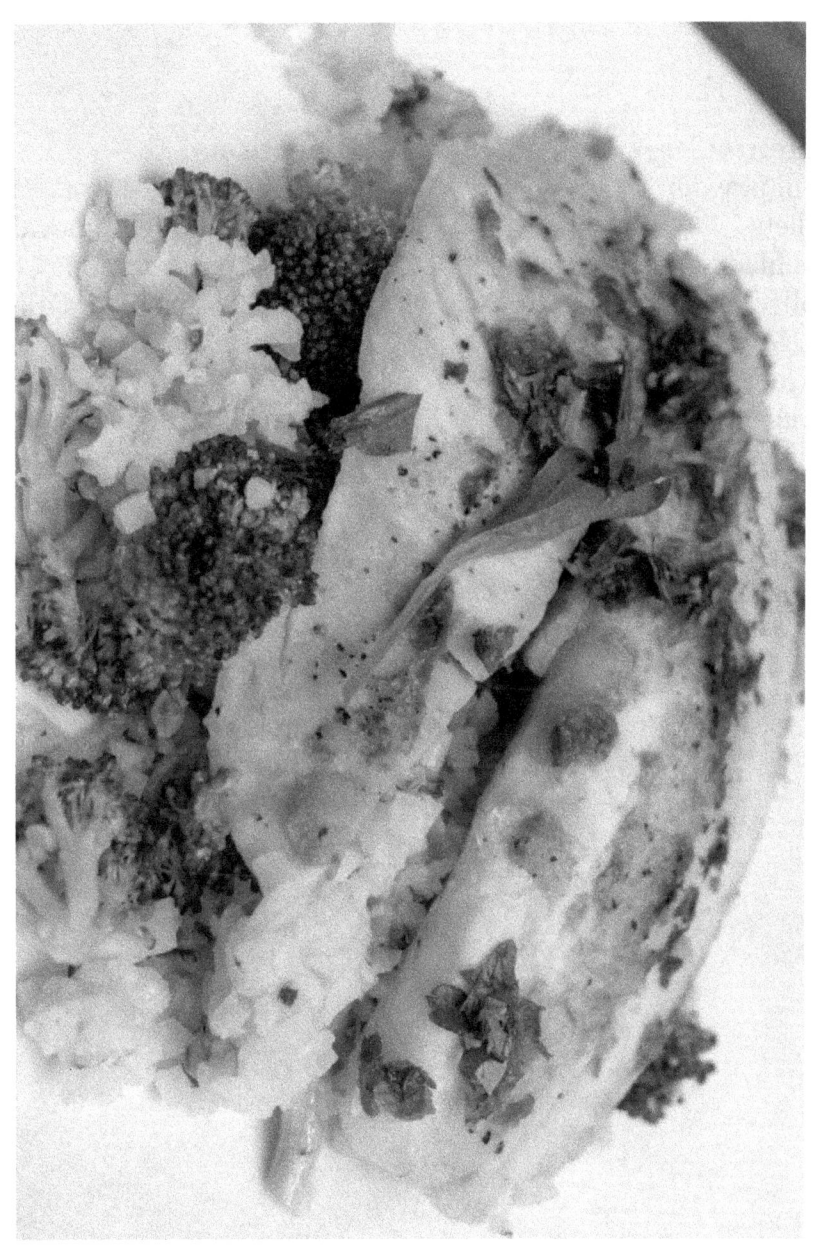

Chili Cod with Chive Sauce

Prep. Time: 25 min
Servings: 2

Ingredients:
1 tsp chili powder
2 cod fillets
Salt and black pepper to taste
1 tbsp olive oil
1 garlic clove, minced
1/3 cup lemon juice
2 tbsp vegetable stock
2 tbsp chives, chopped

Directions:
Preheat oven to 400 F. Rub the cod fillets with chili powder, salt, and pepper and lay in a greased baking dish. Bake for 10-15 minutes. In a skillet over low heat, warm the olive oil and sauté garlic for 1 minute. Add the lemon juice, stock, and chives. Season with salt and pepper and cook for 3 minutes until the sauce slightly reduces. Top the fish with the sauce and serve.

Per serving:
Cal 448; Fat 35g; Net Carbs 6.3g; Protein 20g

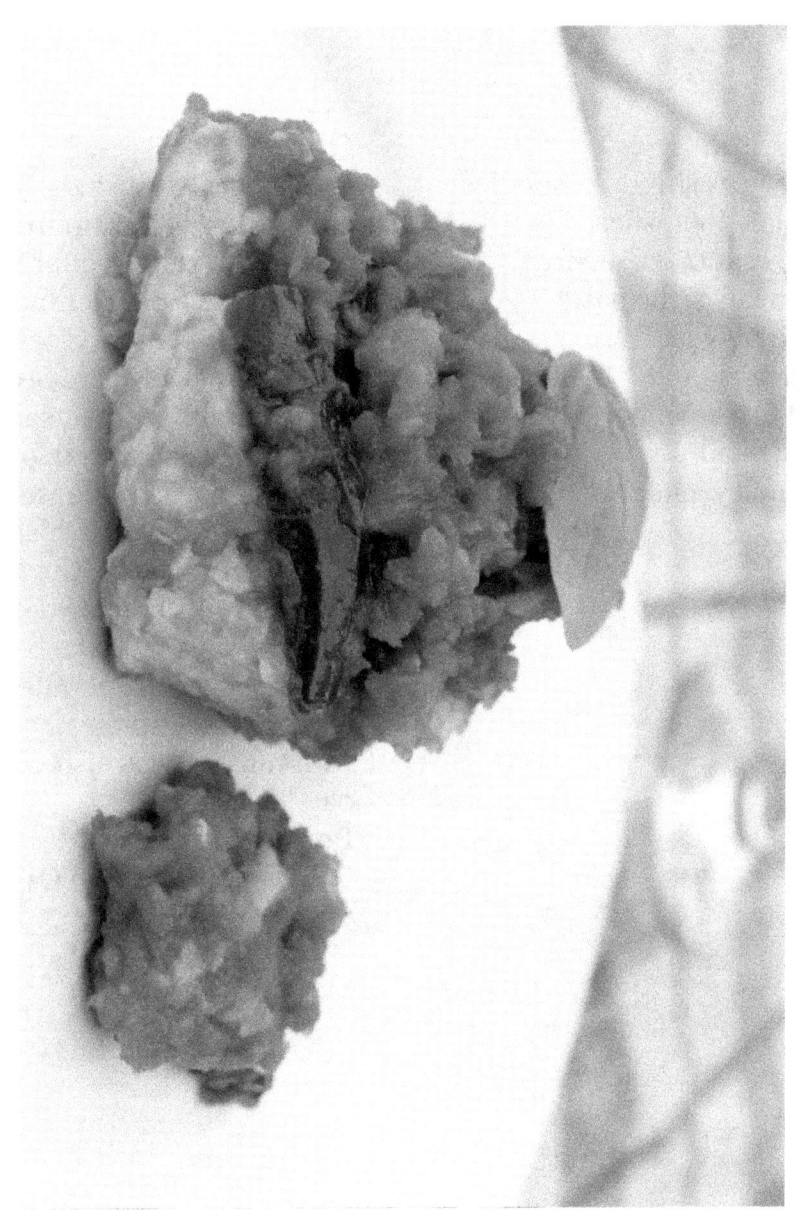

Grilled Tuna with Shirataki Pad Thai

Prep. Time: 20 min
Servings: 2

Ingredients:
½ pack (7-oz) shirataki noodles
1 red bell pepper, sliced
2 tbsp soy sauce, sugar-free
1 tbsp ginger-garlic paste
1 tsp chili powder
2 tuna steaks
Salt and black pepper to taste
2 tbsp olive oil
1 tbsp parsley, chopped

Directions:
In a colander, rinse the shirataki noodles with running cold water. Boil salted water, blanch the noodles for 2/3 minutes.. Drain and set aside. Preheat a grill to medium-high. Season the tuna with pepper, salt and olive oil. Grill covered for 2/3 minutes on each side; set aside covered. In a bowl, whisk soy sauce, ginger paste, the remaining olive oil, chili powder, and 1 tbsp of water. Add the bell pepper and shirataki noodles and toss to coat. Top the noodles with tuna and garnish with parsley to serve.

Per serving:
Cal 287; Fat 16g; Net Carbs 6.8g; Protein 23g

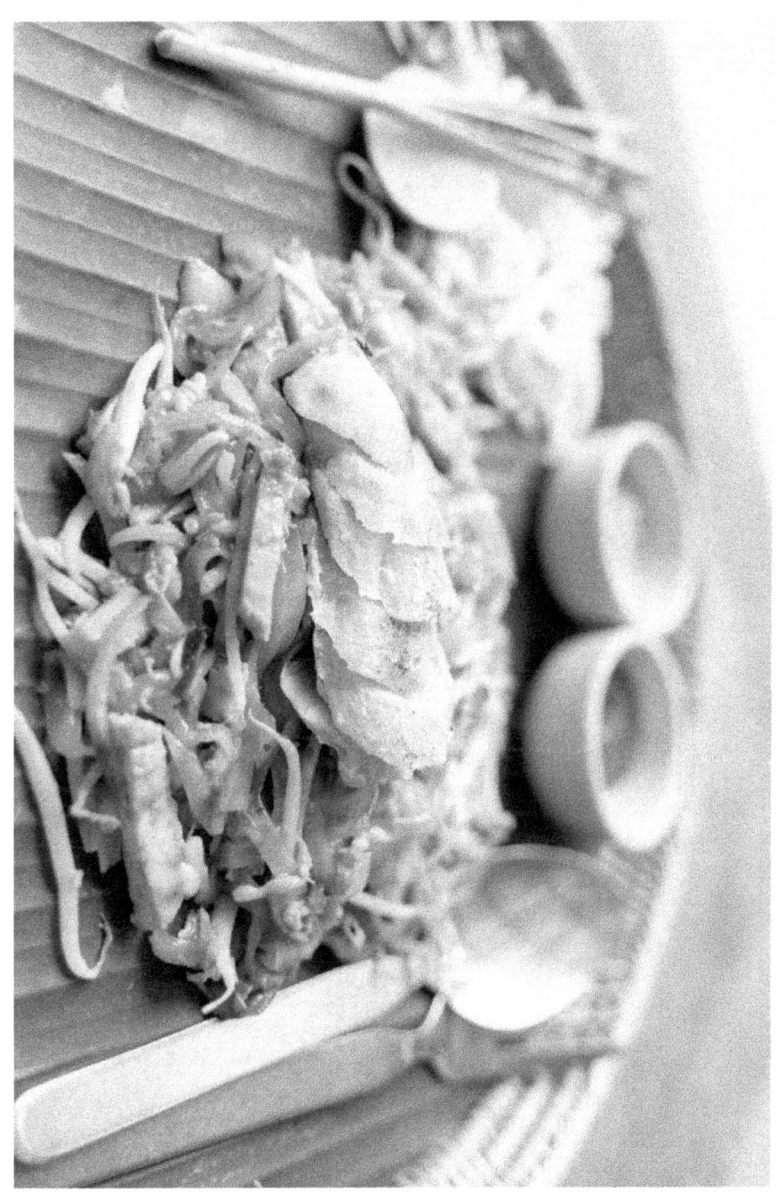

Chapter 6 Snacks, Appetizers & Side Dishes

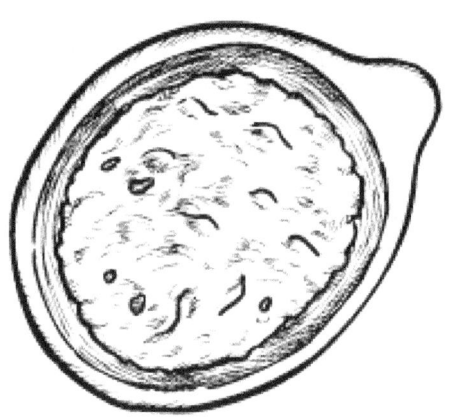

Camembert Bites with Blackberry Sauce

Prep.Time: 40 minutes
Servings: 4

Ingredients:
For the pastry cups
¼ cup butter, cold and crumbled
¼ cup almond flour
3 tbsp coconut flour
½ tsp xanthan gum
¼ tsp cream of tartar
4 tbsp cream cheese, softened
3 whole eggs, unbeaten
1 whole egg, beaten
1 ½ tsp vanilla extract
3 tbsp erythritol
½ tsp salt

For the filling
5 oz Camembert, sliced and cut into 16 cubes
½ cup fresh blackberries
1 tsp butter
1 yellow onion, chopped
3 tbsp red wine
1 tbsp balsamic vinegar
5 tbsp erythritol

Directions:
Preheat oven to 360 F. Turn a muffin tray upside down and lightly grease with cooking spray. In a bowl, mix almond and coconut flours, xanthan gum, and salt. Add in cream cheese, cream of tartar, and butter and mix until crumbly. Stir in erythritol and vanilla extract until mixed. Then, pour in three eggs, one after another, while mixing until formed into a ball. Flatten the dough on a clean flat surface, cover with plastic wrap, and refrigerate for 1 hour. Dust a clean flat surface with almond flour, unwrap the dough, and roll out the dough into a large rectangle. Cut into 16 squares and press each onto each muffin mound on the tray to form a bowl shape. Brush with the beaten egg and bake for 10 minutes. To make the filling, melt butter in a skillet and sauté onion for 3 minutes. Stir in red wine, balsamic vinegar, erythritol, and blackberries. Cook until the berries become jammy and wine reduces, 10 minutes. Set aside. Take out the tray and place cheese cubes in each pastry. Return to oven and bake for 3 minutes. Spoon a tsp each of the blackberry sauce on top. Serve and enjoy!

Per serving:
Cal 369; Net Carbs 4.4g, Fat 32g, Protein 14g

Leafy Greens & Cheddar Quesadillas

Prep.Time: 25 minutes
Servings: 4

Ingredients:
1 tbsp butter, softened
½ cup cream cheese
3 eggs
1½ tsp psyllium husk powder
1 tbsp coconut flour
½ tsp salt
5 oz grated cheddar cheese
1 oz leafy greens

Directions:
Preheat oven to 400 F. In a bowl, whisk the eggs with cream cheese. In another bowl, combine psyllium husk, coconut flour, and salt. Add in the egg mixture and mix until fully incorporated. Let sit for a few minutes. Line a baking sheet with parchment paper and pour in half of the mixture. Bake the tortilla for 7 minutes until brown around the edges. Repeat with the remaining batter. Grease a skillet with the butter and place in a tortilla. Sprinkle with cheddar cheese, leafy greens and cover with another tortilla. Brown each side for 1 minute.

Per serving:
Cal 468; Net Carbs 4g; Fat 40g; Protein 19g

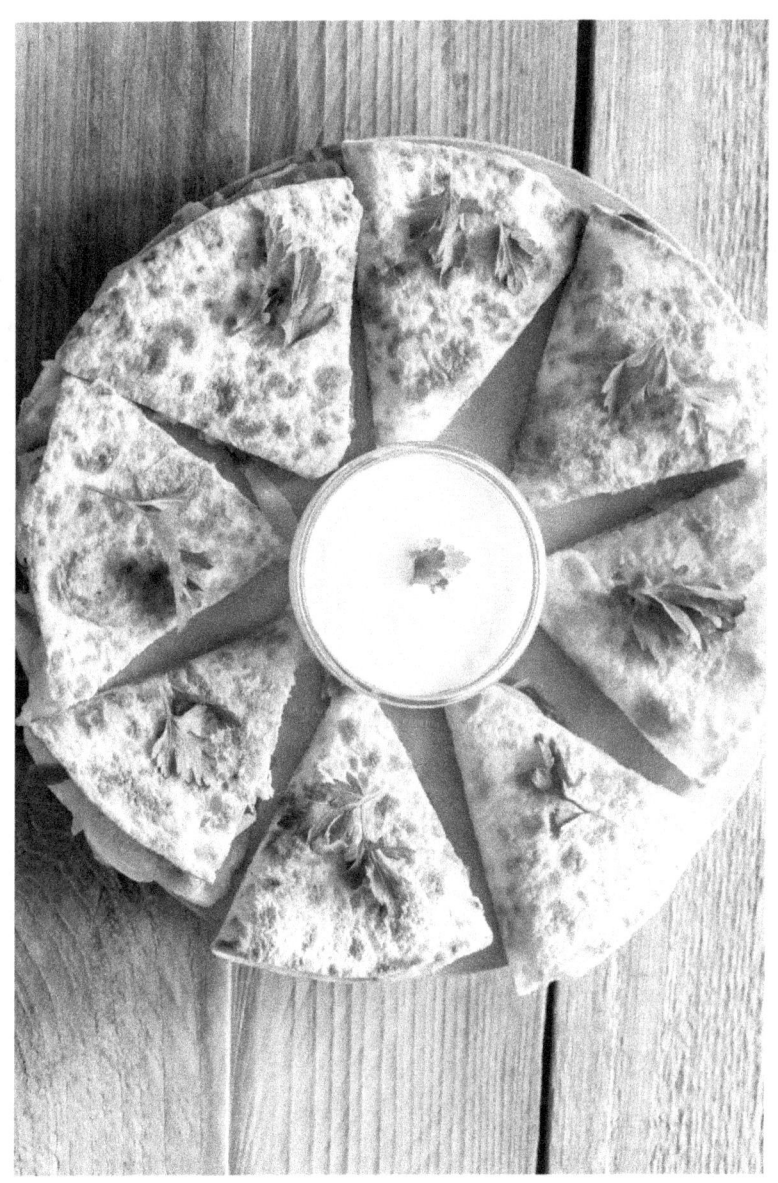

Cheese & Nut Zucchini Boats

Prep.Time: 35 minutes
Servings: 4

Ingredients:
2 medium zucchinis, halved
1 cup cauliflower rice
2 tbsp olive oil
¼ cup vegetable broth
1 ¼ cup diced tomatoes
1 red onion, chopped
¼ cup pine nuts
¼ cup hazelnuts
1 tbsp balsamic vinegar
1 tbsp smoked paprika
1 cup grated Monterey Jack
4 tbsp chopped cilantro

Directions:
Preheat oven to 350 F. Pour cauli rice and broth in a pot and cook for 5 minutes. Fluff the cauli rice and allow cooling. Scoop the flesh out of the zucchini halves and chop the pulp. Brush the zucchini shells with some olive oil. In a bowl, mix cauli rice, tomatoes, red onion, pine nuts, hazelnuts, cilantro, vinegar, paprika, and zucchini pulp. Spoon the mixture into the zucchini halves, drizzle with remaining olive oil, and sprinkle the cheese on top. Bake for 20 minutes until the cheese melts. Serve.

Per serving:
Cal 328; Net Carbs 4.9g; Fat 31g; Protein 12g

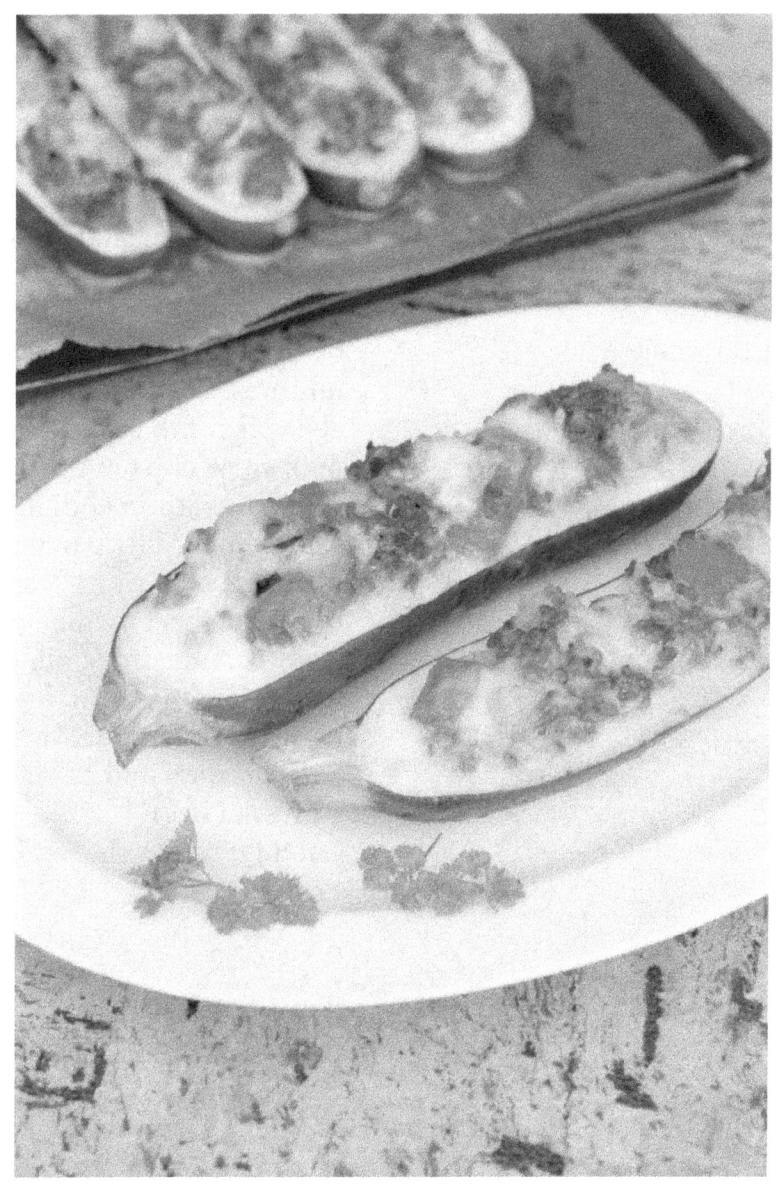

Baked Eggplant Chips with Salad & Aioli

Prep.Time: 30 minutes
Servings: 4

Ingredients:
2 eggplants, sliced
1 egg, beaten
3 ½ oz cooked beets, shredded
3 ½ oz red cabbage, shredded
2 cups almond flour
2 tbsp butter, melted
2 egg yolks
2 garlic cloves, minced
1 cup olive oil
½ tsp red chili flakes
2 tbsp lemon juice
3 tbsp yogurt
2 tbsp fresh cilantro, chopped
Salt and black pepper to taste

Directions:
Preheat oven to 400 F. On a deep plate, mix flour, salt, and pepper. Dip eggplants into the egg, then in the flour. Transfer on a greased baking sheet and brush with butter. Bake for 15 minutes. To make aioli, whisk egg yolks with garlic. Gradually pour in ¾ cup olive oil while whisking. Stir in chili flakes, salt, pepper, 1 tbsp of lemon juice, and yogurt. In a salad bowl, mix beets, cabbage, cilantro, remaining oil, remaining lemon juice, salt, and pepper; toss to coat. Serve the fries with the aioli and beet salad.

Per serving:
Cal 847; Net Carbs 8g; Fat 81g; Protein 26g

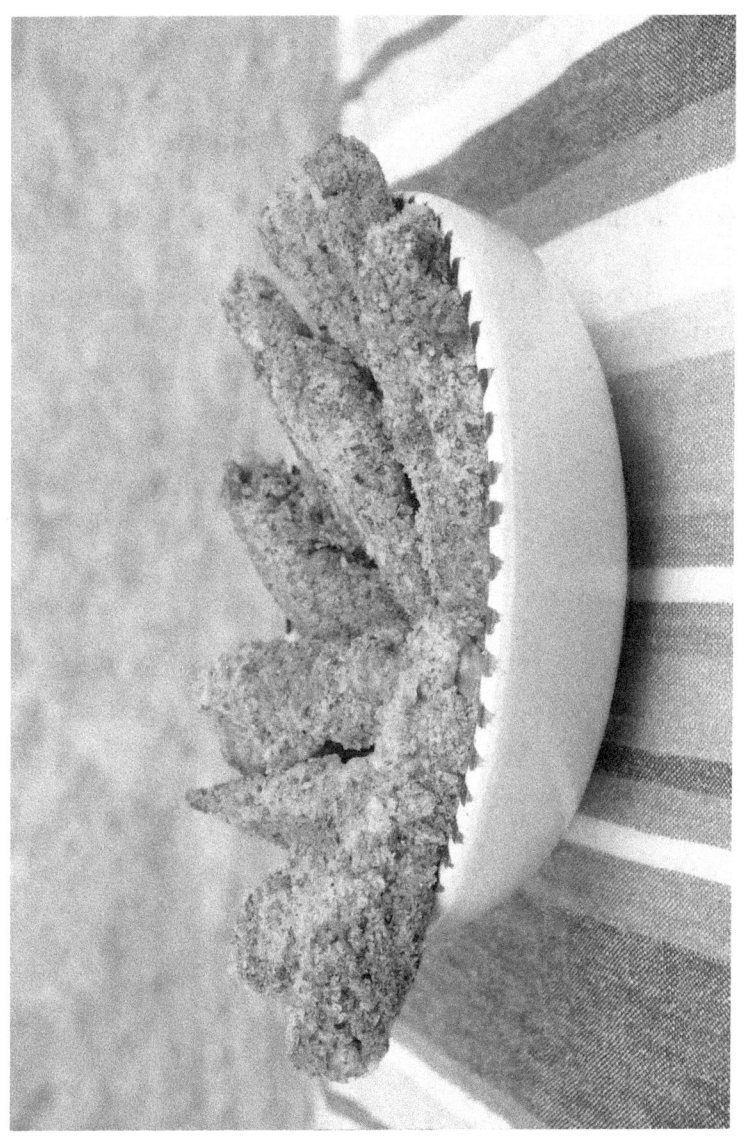

Mushroom & Cheese Lettuce Wraps

Prep.Time: 20 minutes
Servings: 4

Ingredients:
1 iceberg lettuce, leaves extracted
4 oz baby Bella mushrooms, sliced
1 cup grated cheddar cheese
2 tbsp butter
1 lb goat cheese, crumbled
1 large tomato, sliced

Directions:
Warm butter in a skillet over medium/high heat. Add mushrooms and sauté until tender, 6 minutes. Add in goat cheese and cook for 5 minutes, stirring occasionally. Spoon the mixture into the lettuce leaves, sprinkle with cheddar cheese, and top with tomato slices. Serve.

Per serving:
Cal 617; Net Carbs 3g; Fat 52g; Protein 32g

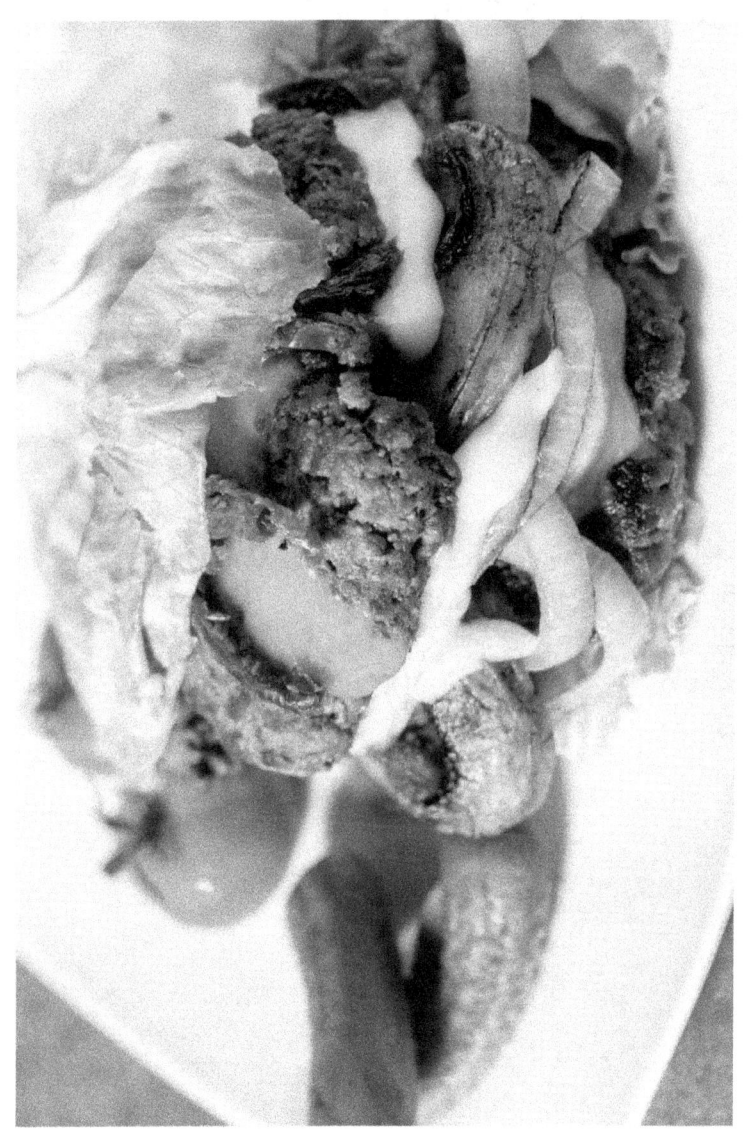

Chapter 7 Desserts, Fruits & Drinks

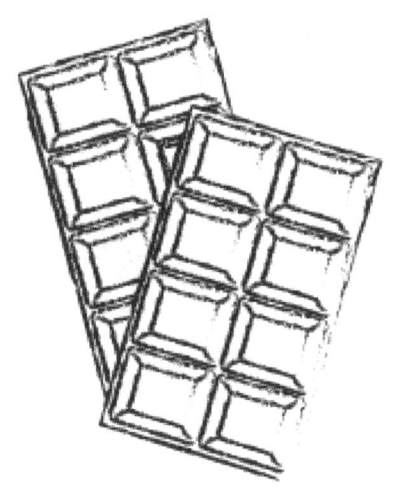

Mascarpone & Strawberry Pudding

Prep. Time: 20 min
Servings: 6

Ingredients:
1 cup mascarpone, softened
2 oz fresh strawberries
1 ¼ cups coconut cream
1 tsp cinnamon powder
1 tsp vanilla extract

Directions:
Put coconut cream into a bowl and whisk until a soft peak forms. Mix in vanilla and cinnamon. Lightly fold in mascarpone and refrigerate for 10 minutes to set. Spoon into serving glasses, top with the strawberries, and serve.

Per serving:
Cal 231; Fat 20g; Net Carbs 3g; Protein 6g

Minty Coconut Parfait with Cranberries

Prep. Time: 15 min
Servings: 4

Ingredients:
1 cup fresh cranberries
2 tbsp hemp seeds
2 cups coconut yogurt
½ lemon, zested
3 mint sprigs, chopped
Sugar-free maple syrup to taste

Directions:
Spoon half of coconut yogurt into 4 serving glasses. Top with cranberries, lemon zest, and hemp seeds. Cover with the remaining coconut yogurt and drizzle with maple syrup. Sprinkle with chopped mint and serve.

Per serving:
Cal 98; Net Carbs 2.9g, Fat 7.8g, Protein 4.7g

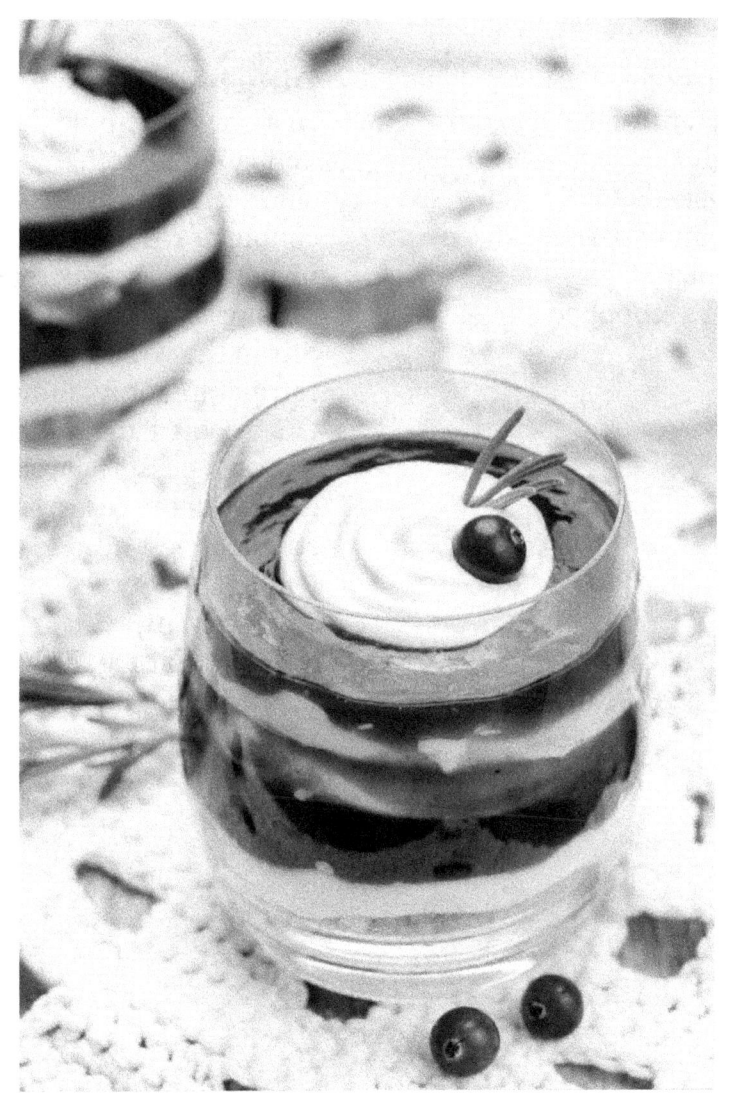

Healthy Chia Pudding With Strawberries

Prep. Time: 20 min
Servings: 4

Ingredients:
1 cup yogurt, full-fat
2 tsp xylitol
2 tbsp chia seeds
1 cup fresh strawberries, sliced
1 tbsp lemon zest
2 mint leaves, chopped

Directions:
In a bowl, combine the yogurt and xylitol together. Add in the chia seeds and stir. Reserve a couple of strawberries for garnish, and mash the remaining ones with a fork until pureed. Stir in the yogurt mixture and refrigerate for 45 minutes. Once cooled, divide the mixture between dessert glasses. Top each with the reserved slices of strawberries, mint leaves, and lemon zest. Serve.

Per serving:
 Cal 187; Fat 11g; Net Carbs 6.3g; Protein 6.7g

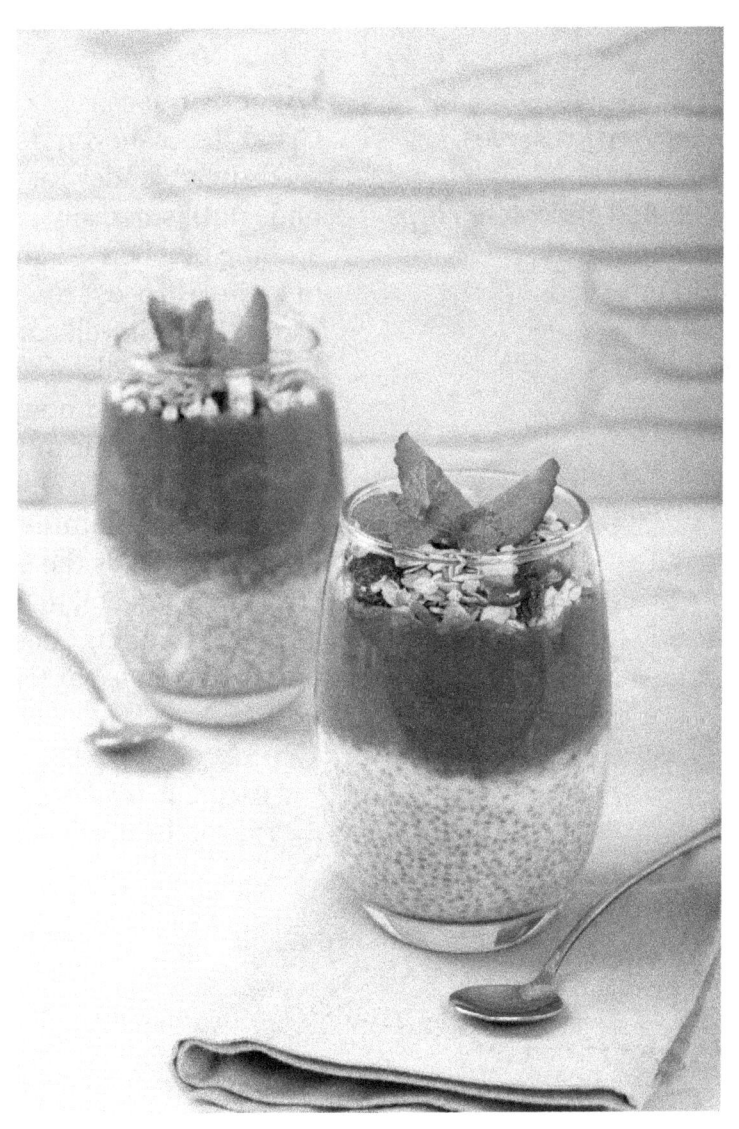

Chocolate Candies with Blueberries

Prep. Time: 15 min
Servings: 4

Ingredients:
1 ½ cups blueberry preserves, sugar-free
10 oz unsweetened chocolate chips
2 cups raw cashew nuts
2 tbsp ground flax seeds
3 tbsp xylitol
3 tbsp olive oil

Directions:
Grind the cashew nuts and flax seeds in a blender for 50 seconds until smoothly crushed; add the blueberries and 2 tbsp of xylitol. Process further for 1 minute until well combined. Form 1-inch balls of the mixture. Freeze for 1 hour or until firmed up. In your microwave, melt the chocolate chips, olive oil, and the remaining xylitol for 95 seconds. Toss the truffles to coat in the chocolate mixture, put on the baking sheet, and freeze up for at least 3 hours.

Per serving:
Cal 253; Fat 18g; Net Carbs 4.1g; Protein 10g

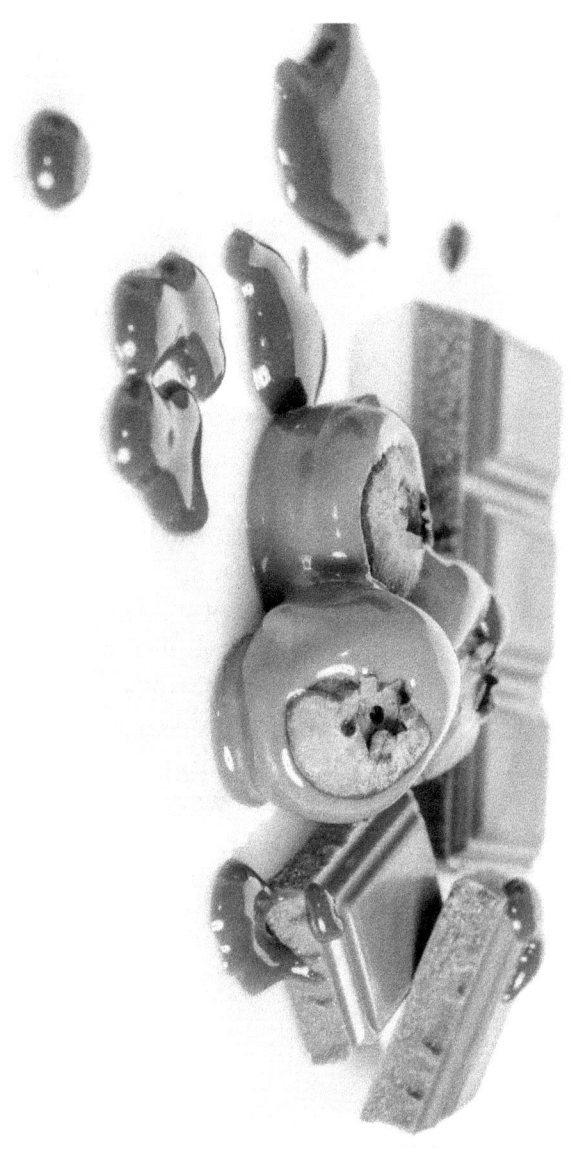

Matcha Brownies with Pistachios

Prep. Time: 30 min
Servings: 4

Ingredients:
4 tbsp Swerve confectioner's sugar
1 tbsp tea matcha powder
¼ cup unsalted butter, melted
A pinch of salt
¼ cup coconut flour
½ tsp baking powder
1 egg
½ cup chopped pistachios

Directions:
Line a square baking dish with parchment paper and preheat the oven to 350 F. In a bowl, pour the melted butter, Swerve sugar, and salt and whisk to combine. Crack the egg into the bowl. Beat the mixture until the egg is incorporated. Pour the coconut flour, matcha, and baking powder into a fine-mesh sieve and sift them into the egg bowl; stir. Stir in the pistachios and pour the mixture into the baking dish to cook for 18 minutes. Remove and slice into brownie cubes.

Per serving:
Cal 243; Fat 22g; Net Carbs 4.3g; Protein 7.2g

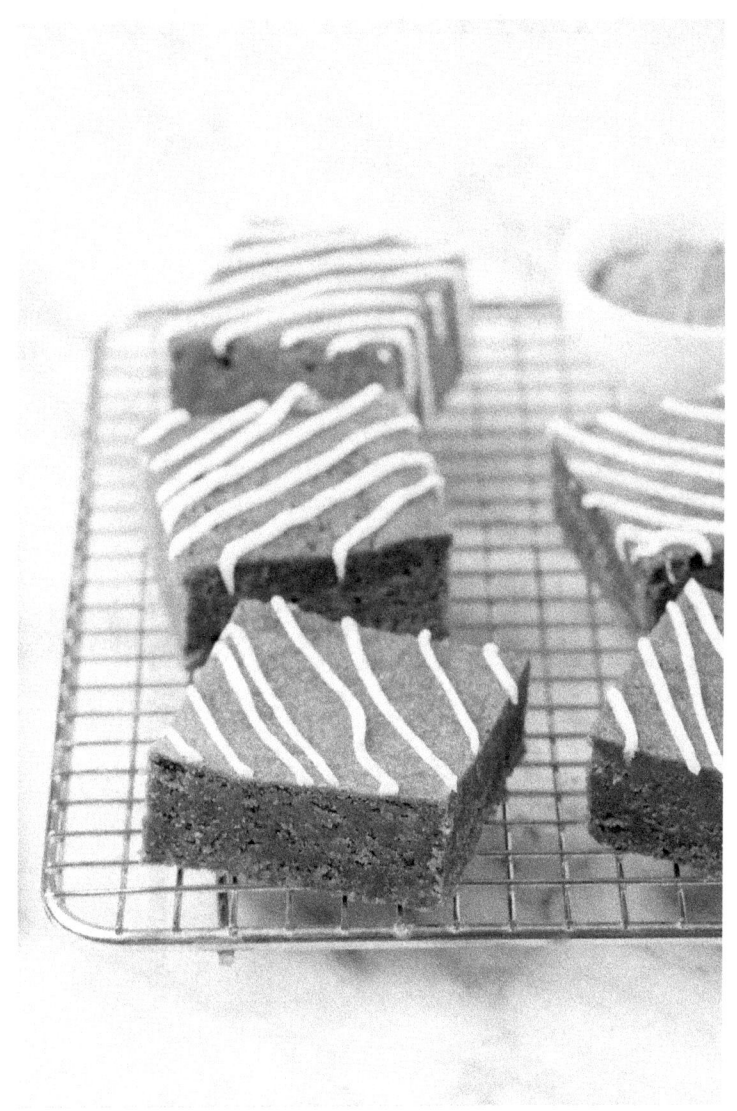

CHAPTER 8 LUNCH

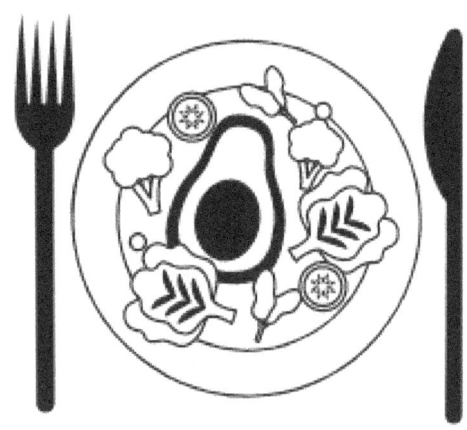

Colorful Turkey Fajitas with Rotini Pasta

Prep.Time: 15 minutes
Servings: 6

Ingredients:
1 ½ lb turkey breast, cut into strips
3 mixed bell peppers, cut diagonally
2 tsp chili powder
1 tsp salt
1 tsp cumin
1 tsp onion powder
1 tsp garlic powder
½ tsp thyme
1 tbsp olive oil
1 red onion, cut into wedges
4 garlic cloves, minced
3 cups chicken broth
1 cup pasta sauce
16 oz rotini pasta
1 cup grated Gouda cheese
½ cup sour cream
½ cup chopped parsley

Directions:
In a bowl, mix chili powder, cumin, garlic powder, onion powder, salt, and thyme. Reserve 1 tbsp of the seasoning. Coat turkey with the remaining seasoning. Warm oil on Sauté. Add in turkey strips and sauté for 5 minutes until browned. Place the turkey in a bowl. Sauté the red onion and minced garlic for 1 minute in the cooker until soft. Mix in salsa and broth and scrape the bottom of any brown bits. Stir in rotini pasta and cover with bell peppers and turkey. Seal the lid and cook for 5 minutes on High Pressure. Do a quick pressure release. Open the lid, sprinkle with shredded gouda cheese and reserved seasoning, and stir well. Divide into plates and top with sour cream. Top with parsley and serve.

Pasta Caprese with Ricotta & Basil

Prep.Time: 15 minutes
Servings: 4

Ingredients:
1 tbsp olive oil
1 onion, chopped
2 garlic cloves, minced
1 tbsp red pepper flakes
2 ½ cups fusilli pasta
1 (15-oz) can tomato sauce
1 cup cherry tomatoes, halved
1 cup water
¼ cup basil leaves
1 tbsp salt
1 cup ricotta, crumbled
2 tbsp chopped fresh basil

Directions:
Warm olive oil on Sauté. Add in garlic, onion and red pepper flakes and cook for 3 minutes until soft. Mix in fusilli, tomatoes, basil, water, tomato sauce, and salt. Seal the lid, and cook on High Pressure for 4 minutes. Release the pressure quickly. Transfer the pasta to a serving platter and top with the crumbled cheese and remaining chopped basil.

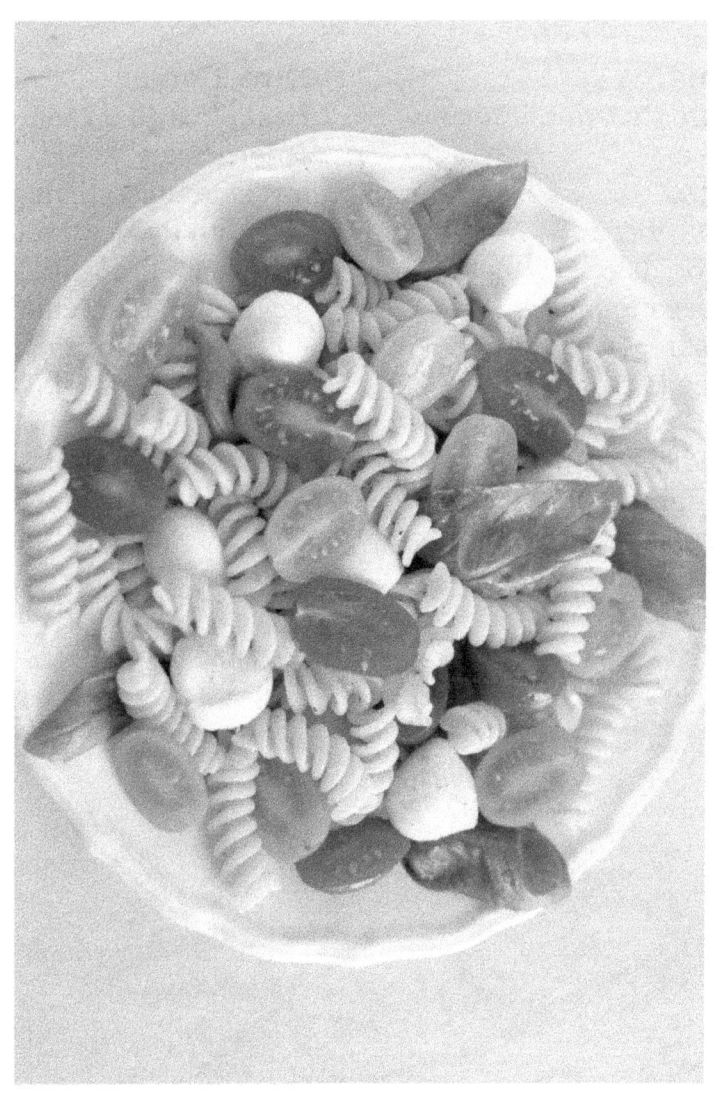

Soup Green Minestrone

Prep.Time: 25 minutes
Servings: 4

Ingredients:
¼ cup grated Pecorino Romano
3 tbsp olive oil
1 onion, diced
1 celery stalk, diced
1 large carrot, diced
14 oz can diced tomatoes
4 oz ziti pasta
1 cup chopped zucchini
1 bay leaf
1 tbsp mixed herbs
¼ tbsp cayenne pepper
Salt and pepper to taste
1 garlic clove, minced
1/3 cup olive pesto pasta

Directions:
Heat olive oil on Sauté. Cook onion, celery, garlic, and carrot for 3 minutes, stirring occasionally until the vegetables are softened. Stir in ziti, tomatoes, 3 cups water, zucchini, bay leaf, mixed herbs, cayenne, pepper, and salt. Seal the lid and cook on High for 4 minutes. Do a pressure release for 10 minutes. Adjust the taste and remove the bay leaf. Ladle the soup into bowls and drizzle the pesto over. Serve topped with Pecorino cheese.

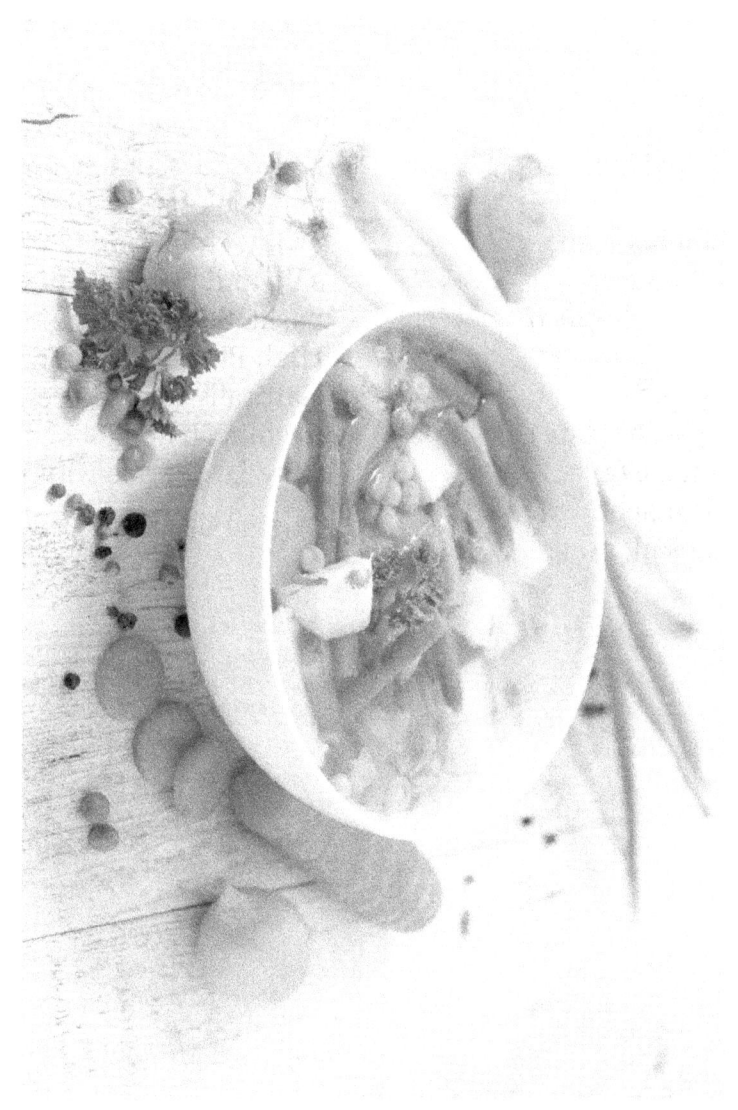

Sausage, Spinach & Tomato Rigatoni

Prep.Time: 30 minutes
Servings: 4

Ingredients:
1 tbsp butter
½ cup diced red bell pepper
1 onion, chopped
3 cups vegetable broth
¼ cup tomato purée
4 sausage links, chopped
½ cup milk
2 tbsp chili powder
Salt and pepper to taste
12 oz rigatoni pasta
1 cup baby spinach
½ cup Parmesan, grated

Directions:
Warm butter on Sauté. Add red bell pepper, onion, and sausage and cook for 5 minutes. Mix in broth, chili, tomato pureé, milk, salt, and pepper. Stir in rigatoni pasta. Seal the lid and cook on High Pressure for 5 minutes. Naturally release pressure. Stir in spinach and let simmer until wilted. Sprinkle with Parmesan and serve.

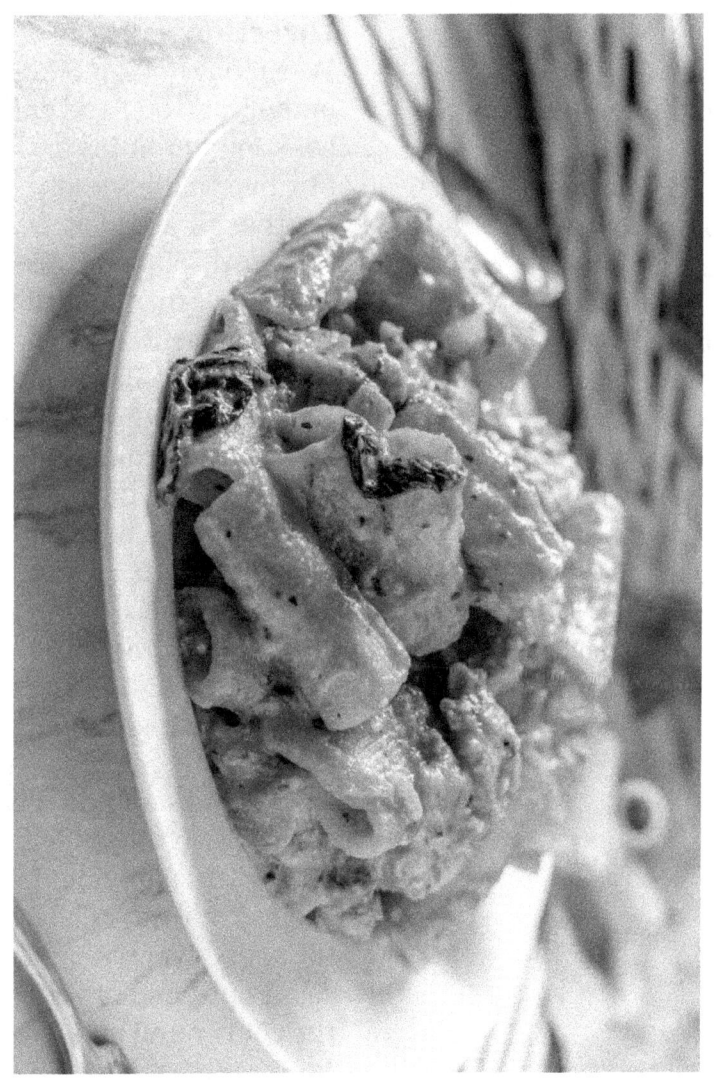

Spinach & Cheese Filled Conchiglie Shells

Prep.Time: 45 minutes
Servings: 6

Ingredients:
¾ cup grated Pecorino Romano cheese
2 cups onions, chopped
1 cup carrots, chopped
3 garlic cloves, minced
3 ½ tbsp olive oil
28-oz can tomatoes, diced
12 oz conchiglie pasta
1 tbsp olive oil for greasing
2 cups ricotta, crumbled
1 ½ cups feta, crumbled
2 cups spinach, chopped
2 tbsp chopped fresh chives
1 tbsp chopped fresh dill
Salt and pepper to taste
1 cup shredded cheddar

Directions:
Warm olive oil on Sauté. Add in onions, carrots, and garlic and cook for 5 minutes until tender. Stir in tomatoes and cook for another 10 minutes. Remove to a bowl. Wipe the pot with a damp cloth, add pasta, and cover with enough water. Seal the lid and cook for 5 minutes on High Pressure. Do a quick release and drain the pasta. Lightly grease olive oil on a baking sheet. In a bowl, combine feta and ricotta cheese. Add in spinach, Pecorino Romano cheese, dill, chives, salt, and pepper and stir. Using a spoon, fill the conchiglie shells with the mixture. Spread 4 cups of the tomato sauce on a baking sheet. Place the stuffed shells over with seam-sides down and sprinkle cheddar cheese on the top. Cover with aluminum foil. Pour 1 cup of water into the cooker and insert a trivet. Lower the baking dish onto the trivet. Seal the lid and cook for 15 minutes on High Pressure. Do a quick release. Take away the foil. Top with the remaining tomato sauce before serving.

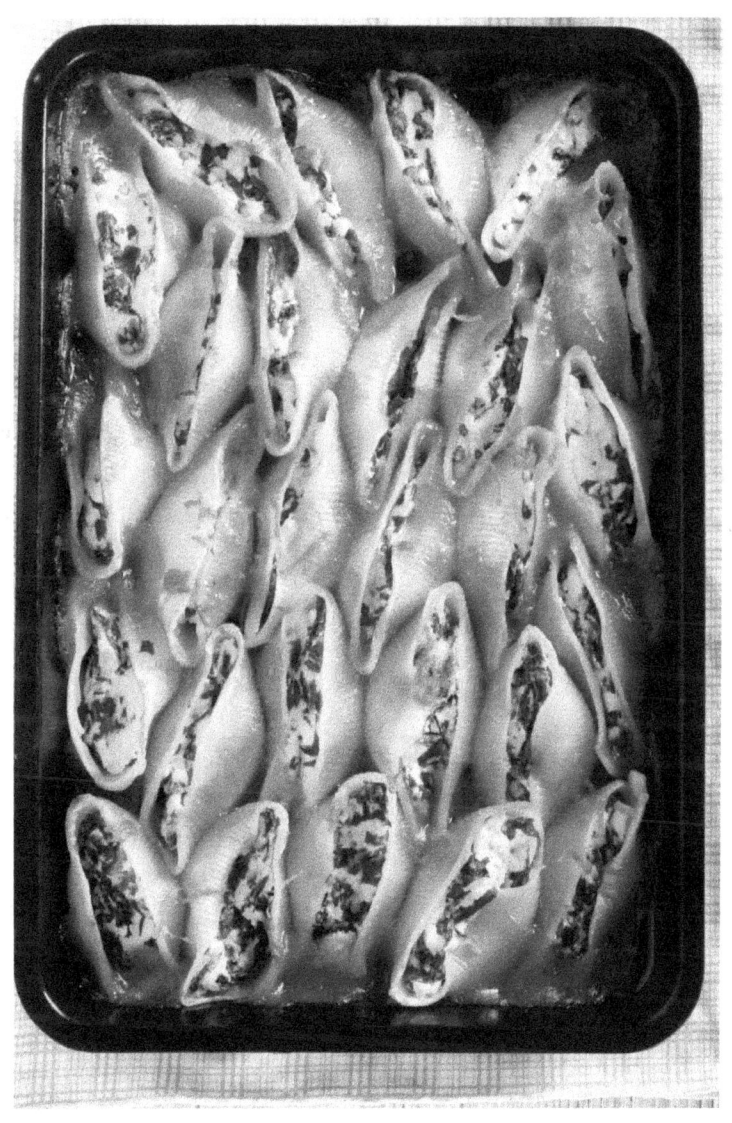

Red Pepper & Chicken Fusilli

Prep.Time: 15 minutes
Servings: 2

Ingredients:
8 oz fusilli pasta
1 cup tomato pasta sauce
1 tbsp paprika
1 red bell pepper, sliced
2 chicken breasts, sliced
2 garlic cloves, chopped
½ tsp Italian seasoning
Salt and red pepper to taste
1 tbsp butter
1 cup Parmesan, grated

Directions:
Stir 1 cup of water, fusilli, and pasta sauce in your Instant Pot. Add in chicken breasts, garlic, red pepper, Italian seasoning, paprika, salt, and pepper and seal the lid. Select Manual and cook for 5 minutes on High. Once over, perform a quick pressure release and unlock the lid. Stir in butter and top with Parmesan cheese to serve.

Creamy Fettuccine with Ground Beef

Prep.Time: 20 minutes
Servings: 6

Ingredients:
10 oz ground beef
1 lb fettuccine pasta
1 cup cheddar, shredded
1 cup fresh spinach, torn
1 medium onion, chopped
2 cups tomatoes, diced
1 tbsp butter
Salt and pepper to taste

Directions:
Melt butter on Sauté. Stir-fry the beef and onion for 5 minutes. Add the pasta. Pour water enough to cover and season with salt and pepper. Cook on High Pressure for 5 minutes. Do a quick release. Press Sauté and stir in the tomatoes and spinach. Cook for 5 minutes. Top with shredded cheddar and serve.

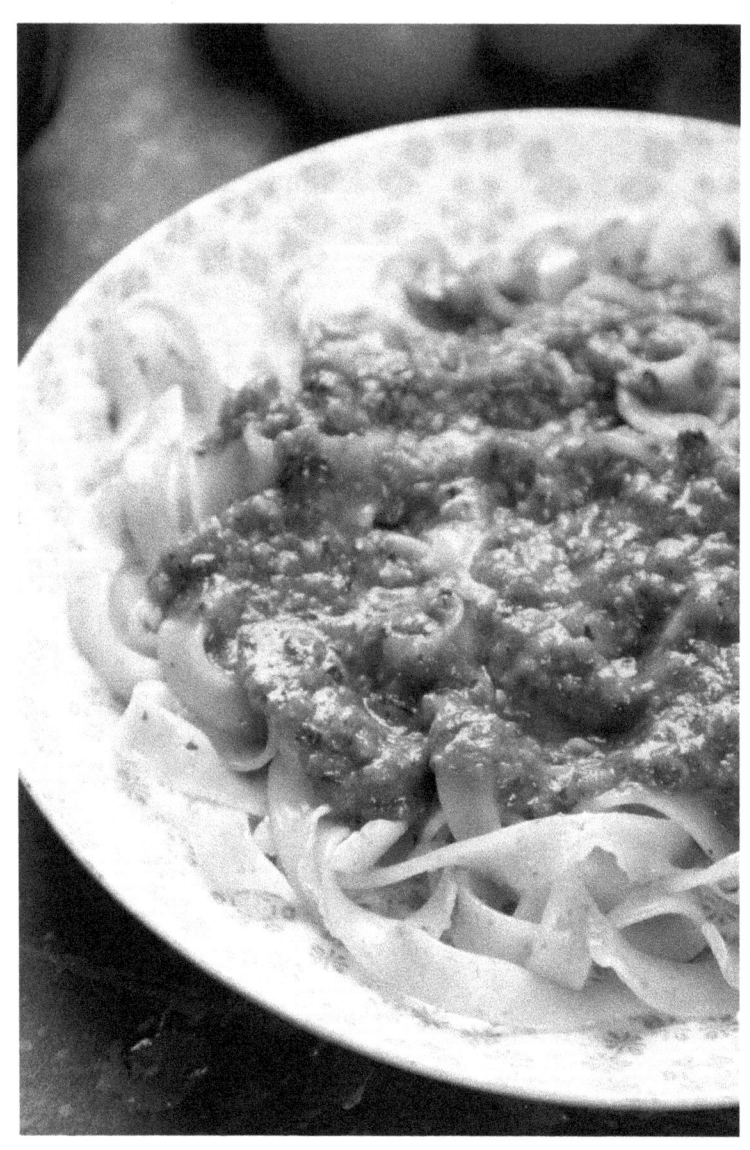

CHAPTER 9 DINNER

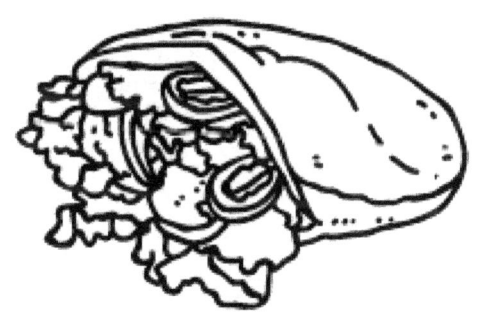

Spinach, Garlic & Mushroom Pilaf

Prep.Time: 45 minutes
Servings: 6

Ingredients:
2 cups button mushrooms, sliced
1 tbsp olive oil
2 cloves garlic, minced
1 onion, chopped
1 cup spinach, chopped
4 cups vegetable stock
2 cups white rice
1 tsp salt
2 sprigs parsley, chopped

Directions:
Select Sauté and heat oil. Add mushrooms, onion, and garlic, and stir-fry for 5 minutes until tender. Mix in rice, stock, spinach, and salt. Cook on High Pressure for 20 minutes, sealing the lid. Release pressure naturally for 10 minutes. Fluff the rice and top with parsley. Serve.

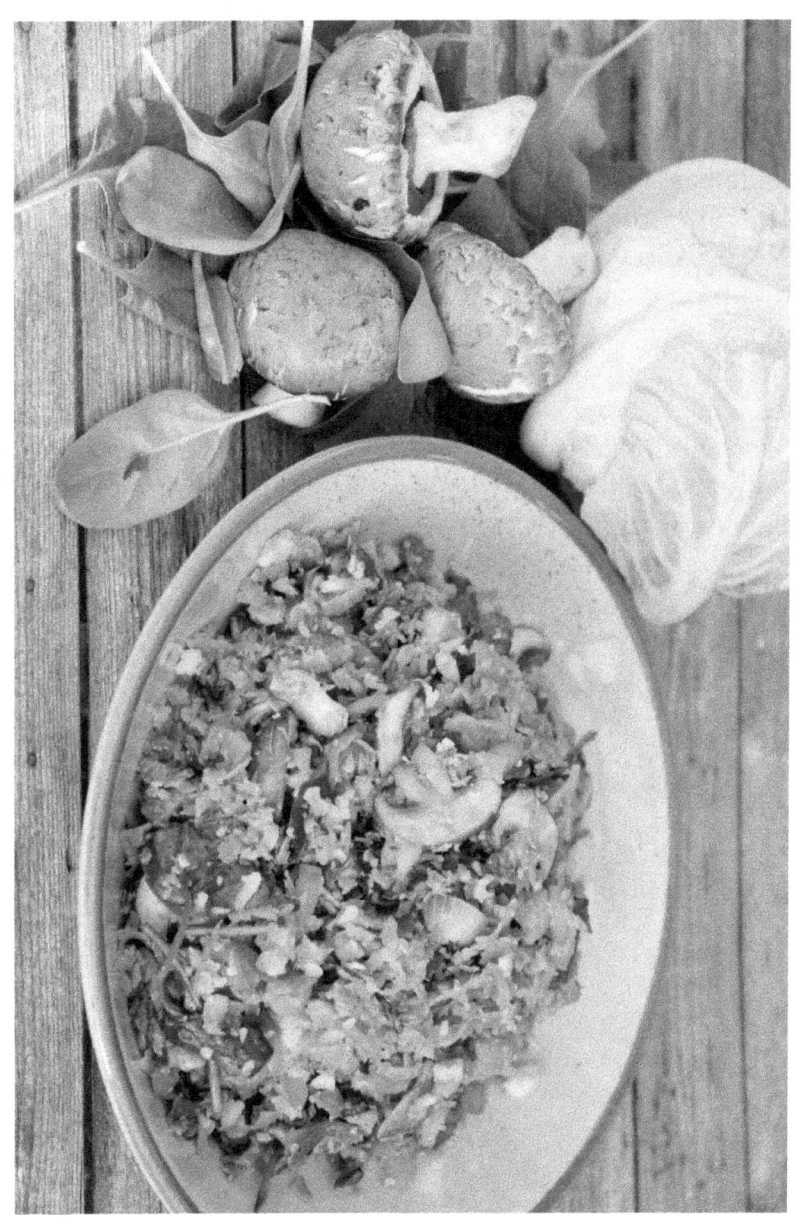

Salmon & Tomato Farfalle

Prep.Time: 20 minutes
Servings: 4

Ingredients:
16 oz farfalle pasta
2 tbsp olive oil
2 garlic cloves, sliced
2 cups tomatoes, diced
¼ tsp chili pepper
¼ tsp oregano
¾ cup red wine
4 oz smoked salmon, flaked
10 green olives, sliced
½ cup Parmesan, grated

Directions:
Warm olive oil in your Instant Pot on Sauté. Add in garlic and cook for 1 minute. Stir in tomatoes, farfalle, chili pepper, 4 cups water, red wine, and oregano. Seal the lid. Select Manual, and cook for 5 minutes on High. Once ready, perform a quick pressure release. Mix in salmon and green olives. Serve sprinkled with Parmesan cheese.

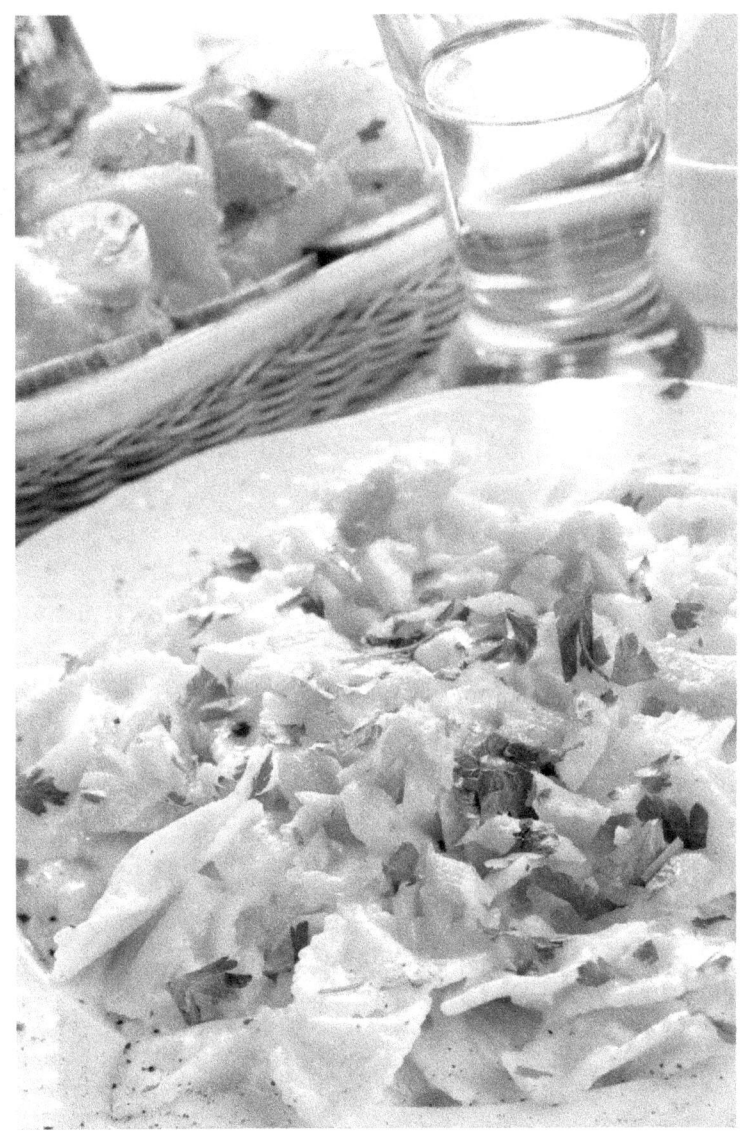

Vegetarian Wild Rice with Carrots

Prep.Time: 30 minutes
Servings: 6

Ingredients:
4 cups vegetable broth
2 carrots, chopped
2 cups wild rice
3 tbsp butter
Zest and juice from 1 lemon
Salt and pepper to taste

Directions:
Add rice, carrots, lemon zest, butter, and broth. Stir, seal the lid, and cook on High Pressure for 12 minutes. Release pressure naturally for 10 minutes. Carefully unlock the lid. Sprinkle salt, lemon juice, and pepper over the rice and use a fork to gently fluff. Serve warm.

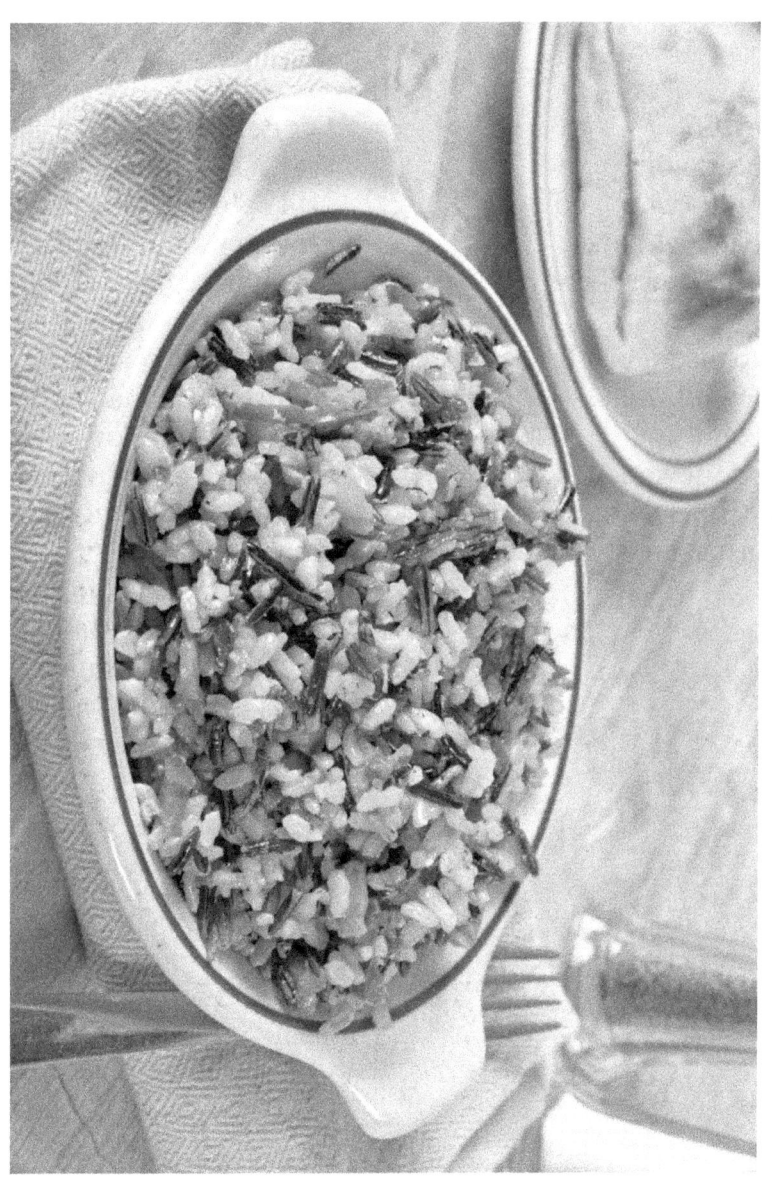

Risotto with Spring Vegetables & Shrimp

Prep.Time: 40 minutes
Servings: 4

Ingredients:
1 tbsp avocado oil
1 lb asparagus, chopped
1 cup spinach, chopped
1 cup mushrooms, sliced
1 cup rice
1 ¼ cups chicken broth
¾ cup coconut milk
1 tbsp coconut oil
1 lb shrimp, deveined
Salt and pepper to taste
¾ cup Parmesan, shredded

Directions:
Warm the avocado oil on Sauté. Add spinach, mushrooms, and asparagus and sauté for 5 minutes until cooked through. Add in rice, coconut milk, and chicken broth as you stir. Seal the lid, press Manual, and cook for 20/22 minutes on High Pressure. Do a quick release. Place the rice on a serving plate. Press Sauté. Heat the coconut oil. Add shrimp and cook for 6 minutes until it turns pink. Set the shrimp over rice and season with pepper and salt. Serve topped with Parmesan cheese.

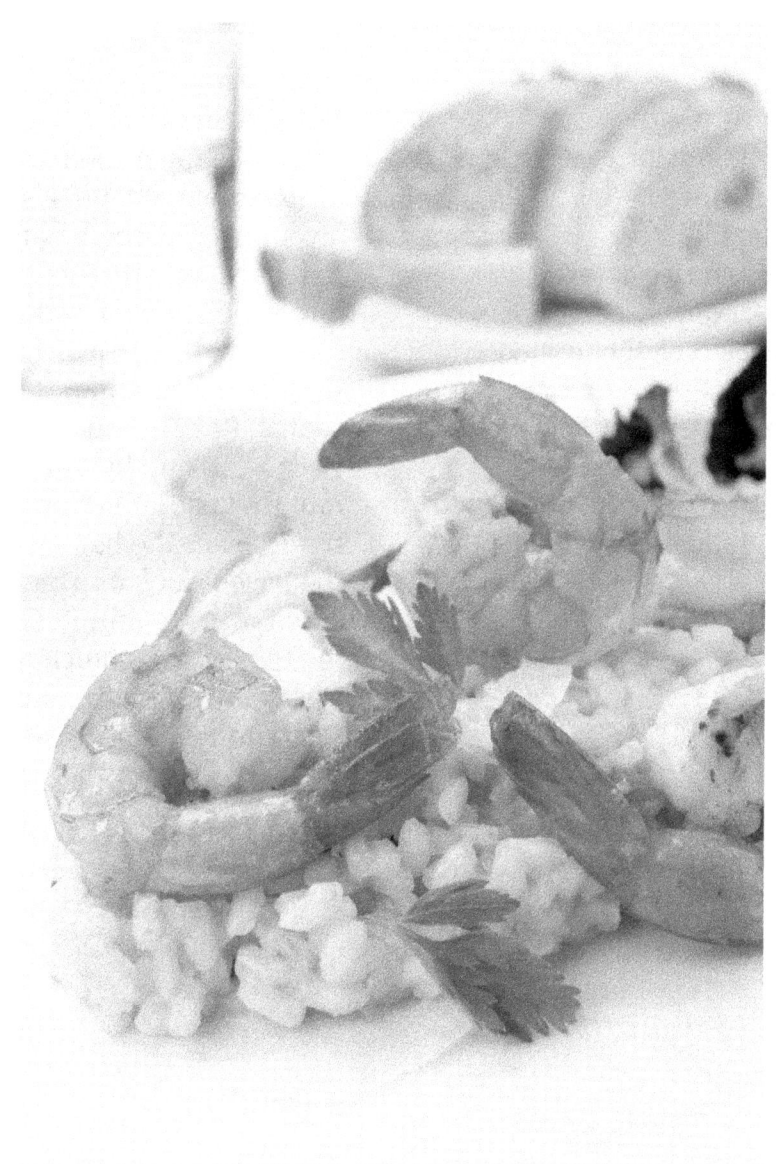

Stuffed Mushrooms with Rice & Cheese

Prep.Time: 30 minutes
Servings: 4

Ingredients:
4 portobello mushrooms, stems and gills removed
2 tbsp melted butter
½ cup brown rice, cooked
1 tomato, chopped
¼ cup black olives, chopped
1 green bell pepper, diced
½ cup feta, crumbled
Salt and pepper to taste
2 tbsp cilantro, chopped
1 cup vegetable broth

Directions:
Brush the mushrooms with butter. Arrange them in a single layer on a greased baking pan. In a bowl, mix the rice, tomato, olives, bell pepper, feta cheese, salt, and black pepper. Spoon the rice mixture into the mushrooms. Pour in the broth.
Pour 1 cup and half of water into the Instant Pot and insert a trivet. Place the baking dish on the trivet. Cook on High Pressure for 10/12 minutes, sealing the lid. Do a quick release. Garnish with fresh cilantro and serve immediately.

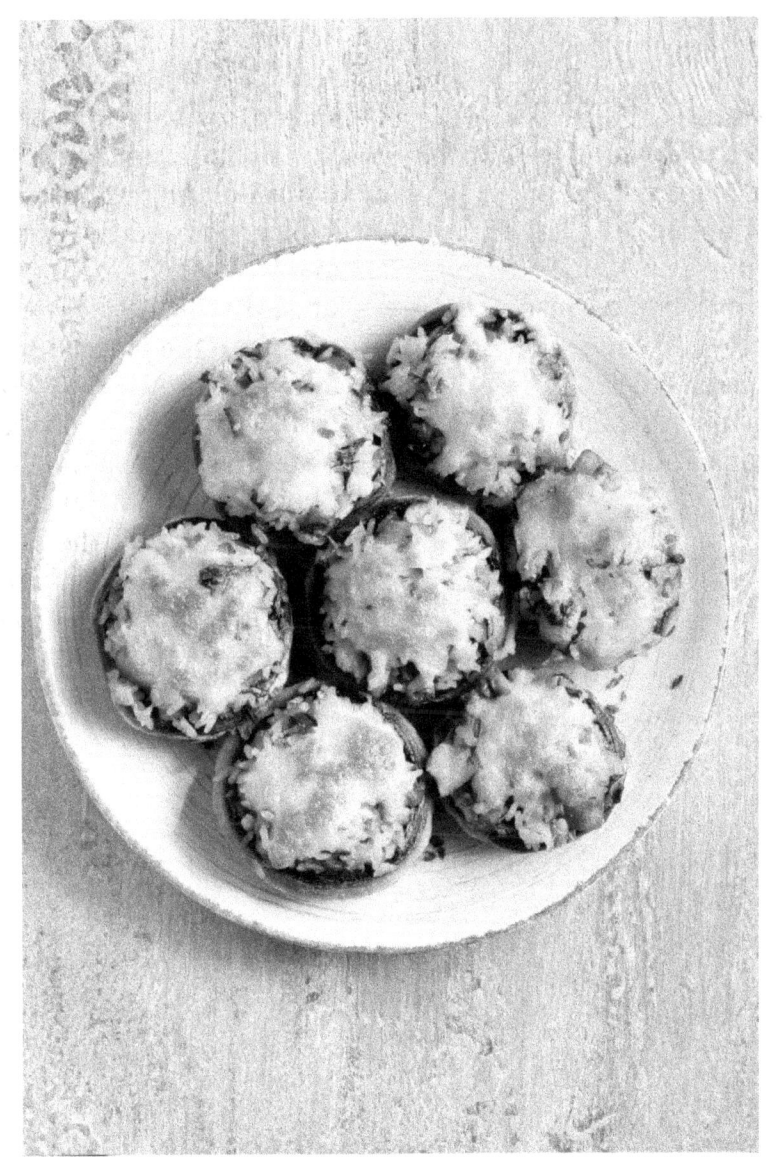

Risotto with Broccoli & Grana Padano

Prep.Time: 30 minutes
Servings: 6

Ingredients:
2 tbsp Grana Padano cheese flakes
10 oz broccoli florets
1 onion, chopped
3 tbsp butter
2 cups carnaroli rice, rinsed
¼ cup dry white wine
4 cups chicken stock
Salt and pepper to taste
2 tbsp Grana Padano, grated

Directions:
Warm butter on Sauté. Stir-fry onion for 3 minutes until translucent. Add in broccoli and rice and cook for 5 minutes, stirring occasionally. Pour wine into the pot and scrape away any browned bits of food from the pan. Stir in stock, pepper, and salt. Seal the lid, press Manual and cook on High for 15 minutes. Release the pressure quickly. Sprinkle with grated Grana Padano cheese and stir well. Top with flaked Grana Padano cheese to serve.

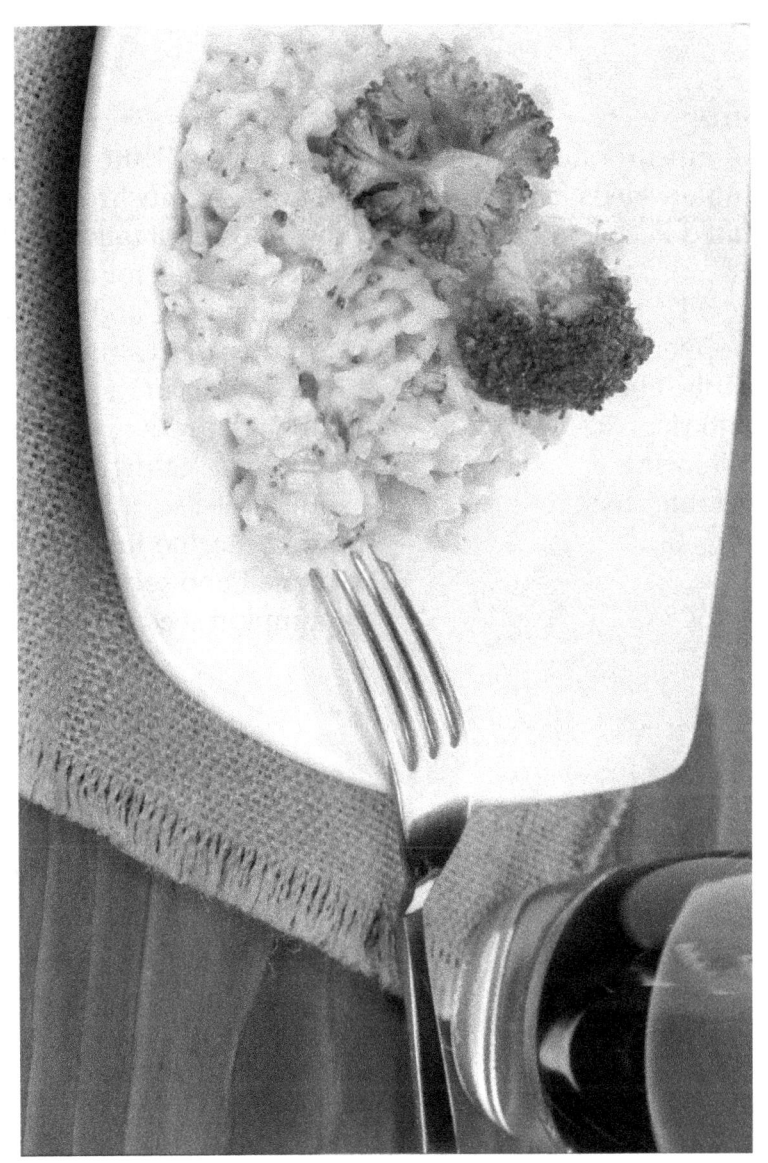

Arugula & Wild Mushroom Risotto

Prep.Time: 30 minutes
Servings: 4

Ingredients:
½ cup wild mushrooms, chopped
4 tbsp pumpkin seeds, toasted
1/3 cup grated Pecorino Romano cheese
2 tbsp olive oil
1 onion, chopped
2 cups arugula, chopped
1 cup arborio rice
1/3 cup white wine
3 cups vegetable stock

Directions:
Heat oil on Sauté and cook onion and mushrooms for 5 minutes until tender. Add the rice and cook for a minute. Stir in white wine and cook for 2-3 minutes until almost evaporated. Pour in the stock. Cook on High Pressure for 10/12 minutes, sealing the lid. Do a quick release. Stir in arugula and Pecorino Romano cheese to melt and serve scattered with pumpkin seeds.

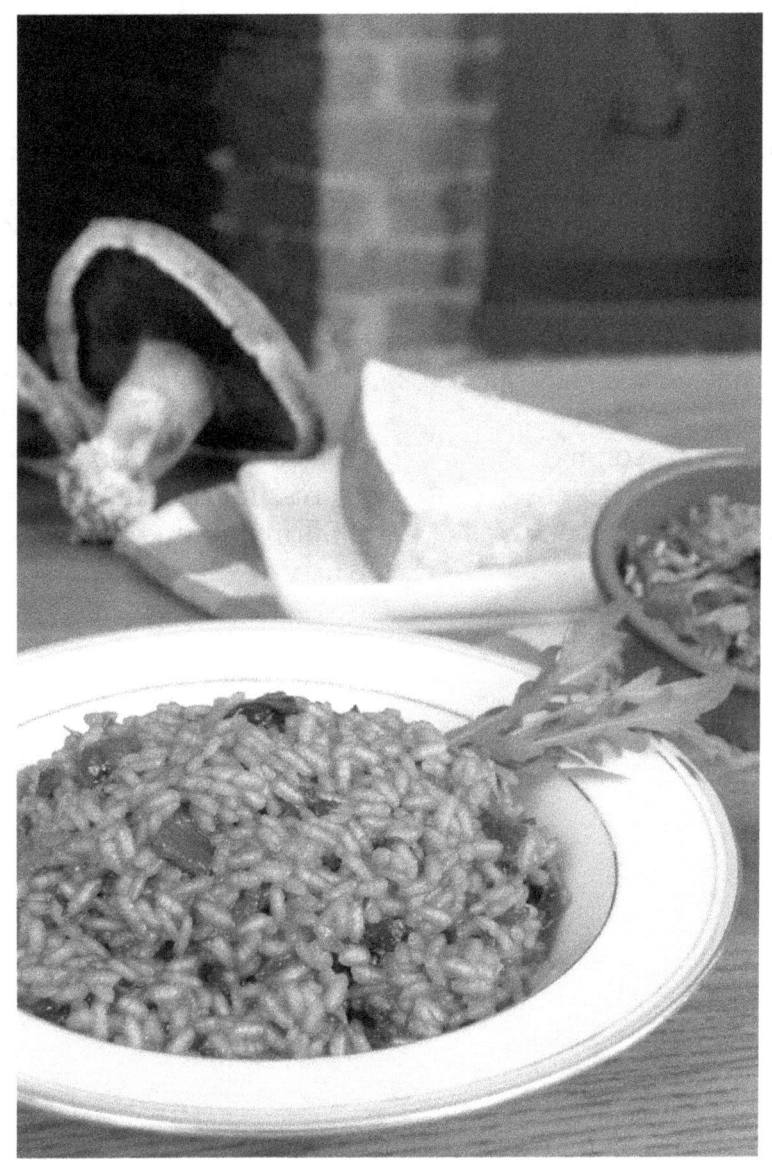

Yummy Mexican-Style Rice & Pinto Beans

Prep.Time: 30 minutes
Servings: 4

Ingredients:
3 tbsp olive oil
1 small onion, chopped
2 garlic cloves, minced
1 serrano pepper, chopped
1 cup rice
1/3 cup red salsa
¼ cup tomato sauce
½ cup vegetable broth
1 tsp Mexican seasoning
16 oz canned pinto beans
1 tsp salt
1 tbsp chopped parsley

Directions:
Warm oil on Sauté and cook onion, garlic, and serrano pepper for 2 minutes, stirring occasionally until fragrant. Stir in rice, salsa, tomato sauce, vegetable broth, Mexican seasoning, beans, and salt. Cook on High Pressure for 10/12 minutes, sealing the lid. Do a natural pressure release for 10 minutes. Sprinkle with fresh parsley and serve.

INDEX RECIPES

A
Arugula & Wild Mushroom Risotto ---------------------------------- 104

B
Baked Eggplant Chips with Salad & Aioli -------------------------- 64
Baked Veggies with Green Salad ----------------------------------- 29
Belgium Waffles with Cheese Spread ------------------------------- 12

C
Camembert Bites with Blackberry Sauce ---------------------------- 59
Chargrilled Zucchini with Avocado Pesto -------------------------- 34
Cheese & Nut Zucchini Boats -------------------------------------- 62
Chicken Salad with Parmesan -------------------------------------- 24
Chili Cod with Chive Sauce --------------------------------------- 54
Chocolate Candies with Blueberries ------------------------------- 74
Classic Egg Salad with Olives ------------------------------------ 20
Colorful Turkey Fajitas with Rotini Pasta ------------------------ 79
Creamy Fettuccine with Ground Beef ------------------------------- 89

F
Feta & Olive Pizza --- 32

G
Ginger Pancakes -- 10
Green Bean & Broccoli Chicken Stir-Fry --------------------------- 42
Green Tuna Traybake -- 49
Grilled Tuna with Shirataki Pad Thai ----------------------------- 56

H
Healthy Chia Pudding With Strawberries --------------------------- 72

J
Jalapeno Waffles with Bacon & Avocado ---------------------------- 9

K
Kale & Broccoli Slaw with Bacon & Parmesan ----------------------- 19

L
Leafy Greens & Cheddar Quesadillas ------------------------------- 60

M
Marinated Fried Chicken -- 46
Mascarpone & Strawberry Pudding ---------------------------------- 69

Matcha Brownies with Pistachios — 76
Minty Coconut Parfait with Cranberries — 70
Mushroom & Cheese Lettuce Wraps — 66

P

Paprika Chicken & Pancetta in a Skillet — 40
Pasta Caprese with Ricotta & Basil — 80
Peanut Butter & Pastrami Gofres — 16

R

Red Pepper & Chicken Fusilli — 88
Risotto with Broccoli & Grana Padano — 102
Risotto with Spring Vegetables & Shrimp — 98
Roasted Pepper with Tofu — 30
Roasted Pork Stuffed with Ham & Cheese — 44

S

Salmon & Tomato Farfalle — 94
Sausage, Spinach & Tomato Rigatoni — 84
Shirataki Fettucine with Salmon — 50
Smoked Mackerel Lettuce Cups — 26
Soup Green Minestrone — 82
Spinach & Brussels Sprout Salad — 22
Spinach & Cheese Filled Conchiglie Shells — 86
Spinach & Feta Cheese Pancakes — 14
Spinach, Garlic & Mushroom Pilaf — 92
Stuffed Mushrooms with Rice & Cheese — 100

T

Tilapia Tortillas with Cauliflower Rice — 52

V

Vegetarian Wild Rice with Carrots — 96

W

Walnut & Feta Loaf — 36

Y

Yummy Mexican-Style Rice & Pinto Beans — 106

Z

Zucchini & Bell Pepper Chicken Gratin — 39

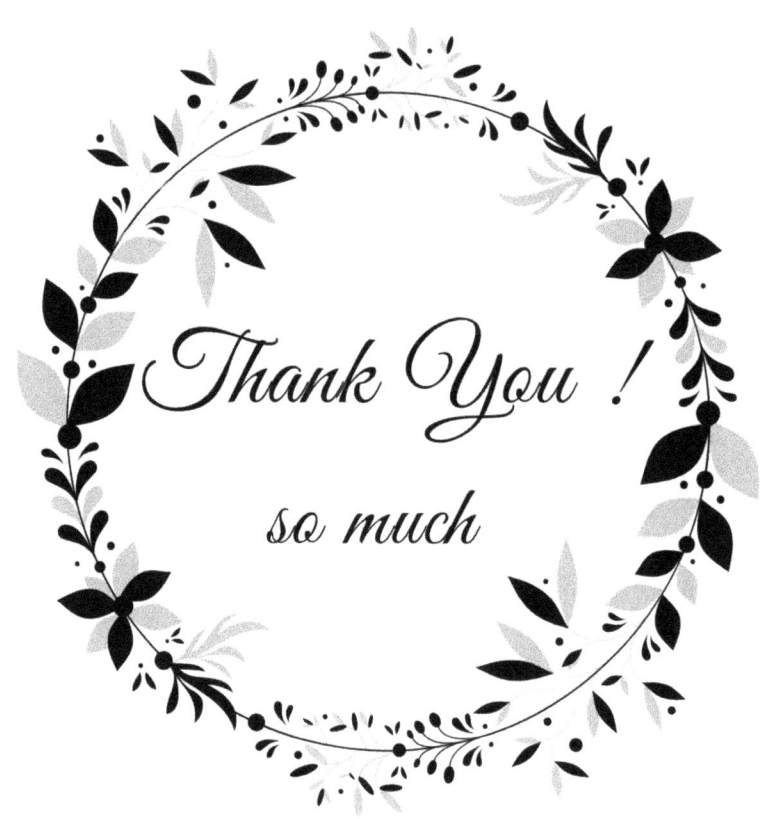

CPSIA information can be obtained
at www.ICGtesting.com
Printed in the USA
BVHW091333210621
610125BV00005B/1473